T0173684

Life in the Balance

'A remarkably honest memoir of a life spent pulling people back from death, with stories ranging from the fascinating to the terrifying'

Adam Kay, author of *This is Going to Hurt*

'If Jim Down is as good a doctor as he is a writer, his patients are in very safe hands. Whether treating famous Russian spies, the victims of terrorist attacks, or people taken close to death by Covid, he shows us what it's really like to care for those who are clinging to life, and describes with unflinching honesty the toll that working in intensive care can take on his own mental health, and that of his colleagues'

Alastair Campbell

'Beautifully written, witty and heartbreaking. A reminder to do everything we can to help our extraordinary NHS'

Olivia Colman

'*Life in the Balance* brims with the wonder, trauma and magic of medicine. Jim Down is a consummate storyteller whose tales of life and death in the ICU are riveting. I loved this book'

Dr Rachel Clarke, author of *Breathtaking*

'Spies, terror, personal crisis, resolution and redemption; *Life in the Balance* really has it all . . . A hilarious, beautiful book, I was sincerely moved'

Dr Chris van Tulleken

'A page-turning gritty biography of a top intensive care doctor's experiences of the front line in London. Transport yourself into the angst-ridden, terrifying and at times hilarious world of the trainee doctor of the 1990s. A cross between *This is Going to Hurt* and *Do No Harm*'

Dr Andrew Jenkinson

'There are so many compelling stories here. Jim Down is as remarkable a writer as he is a doctor. It is like being by the patient's bedside in critical care – but more than that you are inside Jim's head as he struggles with ethical as well as medical dilemmas. What comes across most strongly is his humanity. If I'm ever in ICU I hope he's my consultant'

Fergus Walsh, Medical Editor, BBC

'Whoever you are, you should read this book. One in five of you will, at some point, need a Jim'

Hugh Montgomery, Professor of Intensive Care Medicine, University College London

'Medical students should read this. Young doctors should read this. Patients should read this. Having read it, I have no idea how Dr Down found the time to write it!'

Sir Richard Stilgoe

Life in the Balance

A Doctor's Stories of Intensive Care

JIM DOWN

VIKING
an imprint of
PENGUIN BOOKS

VIKING

UK | USA | Canada | Ireland | Australia
India | New Zealand | South Africa

Viking is part of the Penguin Random House group of companies
whose addresses can be found at global.penguinrandomhouse.com

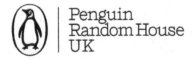

First published 2023
002

Copyright © Jim Down, 2023

The moral right of the author has been asserted

Set in 12/14.75 pt Bembo Book MT Pro
Typeset by Jouve (UK), Milton Keynes
Printed and bound in Great Britain by Clays Ltd, Elcograf S.p.A.

The authorized representative in the EEA is Penguin Random House Ireland,
Morrison Chambers, 32 Nassau Street, Dublin D02 YH68

A CIP catalogue record for this book is available from the British Library

ISBN: 978–0–241–50638–7

www.greenpenguin.co.uk

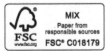

For Tish, Edie and Tom

Contents

1. Origins

'He's got what?'

'Gram negative rods in his blood. Sorry, I meant to say this morning.'

'Jesus, Jim! When did you find out?'

'They bleeped me, I was . . .' (I'd been in the toilet.) 'I didn't have a pen and then it slipped my mind. He's on antibiotics . . .'

'We stopped them – the oral Amoxil from the GP, and now his blood pressure's . . . ?'

'Eighty. According to the staff nurse, but she's rechecking it.'

'You've got good IV access?'

'We did, but it's just tissued –'

'I've got two chest pains here, I can't leave –'

'I'll go and try again.'

'He needs fluids and antibiotics – Augmentin and gent IV.'

'Yup.'

'Have you called ICU?'

'I'll phone them now.' I paused. 'Sorry, Sophie.'

I turned away before she could say anything else and ran back down the 200-metre corridor to Murray ward.

It was September 1994, but I can still remember the miserable feeling of fear, panic, guilt and embarrassment as if it were yesterday. I've felt it many times since. I'd been a doctor for just over a month and I was the medical house officer in a large university teaching hospital in Bristol.* I was sharing a house with

* All newly qualified doctors had to complete six months as a medical house officer, the most junior member of the team (admitting all the patients with

four medical-school mates, and in many ways we were still living a student life. We spent too much time in the pub, ate very few vegetables and washed up only sporadically, but we weren't students any more, we were doctors. We were the lowest of the low in the medical hierarchy, 'house plants', yet to register fully with the General Medical Council (GMC), but we'd got the title and were in equal measure giddy with the achievement and terrified. In the hospital, instead of being students who were a nuisance and 'in the way' all the time, we had a role and an iota of respect. Unfortunately, with that came the expectation that we'd know stuff, be able to do things and, worst of all, make decisions. No longer could we just peruse blood tests or X-rays with vague academic interest: now we had to act on them. We had to decide whether a result was important or urgent and then proceed accordingly, and I'd just made my first big mistake. I'd failed to recognize a 'sick' patient and now his life was in danger.

He was a fifty-five-year-old man called Petros whom we'd admitted in the early hours of that Saturday morning. Our 'firm', consisting of a consultant, a registrar, a senior house officer (SHO) and me, were on call for the weekend – Friday morning until Monday evening. The SHO, Sophie, and I would not leave the hospital in that time, so we were thirty hours into an eighty-hour shift.*

---

heart attacks, pneumonias, strokes, etc.) and six months as a surgical house officer (the equivalent, but admitting those patients who might need an operation). At the end of this, catastrophic incompetence excepted, they were granted full registration with the GMC.

* In the 1960s the junior doctors lived on the hospital campus. Their social lives were usually based around the hospital and they were on call for their patients every other night, but they were looked after. My father remembers handing his bleep over to a porter before dinner was served at 7.07 precisely

Petros had come in feeling generally unwell, with some non-specific pain in his lower chest, lethargy, nausea and vomiting. He didn't look great, but his blood pressure was OK and his oxygen saturations, although a bit low initially, picked up with supplemental oxygen.* Petros's heart was batting along a bit fast, but he was frightened and he'd just been sick so that seemed an adequate explanation to me. His GP had been treating a chest infection for a few days, but his chest sounded clear when I listened to it with my shiny new stethoscope, except for a few

---

in the boardroom of the Royal Brompton Hospital. One of the junior doctors carved the joint, beer was served with the meal and, should the wards require his services, the porter would approach discreetly and whisper in his ear. Other hospitals were less predictable and busier but he expected to sleep for at least part of the night, because he was responsible for a small group of patients and the emergency interventions were limited. Thirty years later, when I qualified, I was only on call once every four nights and weekends, but although roast dinner and beer had gone and the nocturnal workload had increased significantly it was still an on-call system. I worked the days before and after my nights and retired to my on-call room when I could. Over the subsequent ten years the nights continued to get busier and it became apparent that this system was not sustainable (or legal under European Working Time directives) so on-call rotas were gradually replaced by shift work and the on-call rooms were removed. Many people rue the loss of the old system, particularly missing the teamwork of the 'firms', the loss of continuity of patient care and the camaraderie of the 'good old days', but the truth is that as the pressures on the NHS increased a different approach was required. There were positives about the old system and if those on-call rooms could speak they'd have some tales to tell but, despite the Tory cuts, I'd rather be a patient in today's NHS – and those eighty-hour shifts were awful.
* The clothes peg they put on your finger in the emergency department measures the percentage of haemoglobin that is saturated with oxygen in your arterial blood. Haemoglobin is the molecule that carries the majority of oxygen around the circulation. When fully oxygenated it gives the blood its red colour, when deoxygenated the blood turns ominously blue.

crepitations at the lung bases,* and his temperature was only mildly elevated. He did not display the clear-cut diagnostic criteria that the medical textbooks would have us expect, but our money was on his heart or possibly a blood clot to the lungs. The nausea and vomiting could be a viral stomach bug, a side-effect of the antibiotics or just all part of being unwell. We'd admitted him, given him supplementary oxygen and some diuretic to offload fluid and ordered a battery of blood and urine tests, an ECG and a chest X-ray. My job was to chase up all the results, interpret them and report back to my seniors, who at that stage were not overly concerned. His ECG was reassuring – no signs of a heart attack – his chest X-ray was 'a bit fluffy' but not too bad,† and his initial blood results were only mildly abnormal so, despite the fact that his heart was still going a little fast and his blood pressure lowish, as dawn broke, he slipped down the pecking order of my inexperienced medical brain. I had two new patients who'd just arrived and needed 'clerking' (the initial admission and assessment) and I was knackered and starving.

'Positive blood culture on your man Mr Bouras,' the lab technician had informed me, when (having left the toilet), I'd eventually found a free corridor phone to answer my bleep. 'Gram negative rods, grew within eight hours.'

In those days there were no mobile phones and, as well as looking up urgent results on a primitive computer, we used to

---

* Crepitations, often shortened to 'creps' or 'crackles', describes a noise in the chest that sounds like a crisp packet being scrunched. It implies that the lung air spaces have fluid in them and are opening and closing when the patient breathes in and out.

† Chest X-ray interpretation is hard! The two-dimensional representation of a three-dimensional space creates many subtleties and ambiguities and over- or under-interpretation is very common.

receive them as a stack of paper slips (sent manually from the lab), that we read through and then initialled as 'reviewed'. The vast majority were unremarkable or of limited significance, and although I knew it was not normal to have bacteria in your blood, I failed to register the importance of what I'd just heard. (It was also not normal to be bleeped with a routine result, but the implications of that passed me by as well. I just assumed that the lab technician was being particularly conscientious and helpful.)

Several areas of the body always contain bacteria – the mouth, colon and skin being good examples – and living in balance with the right bacteria in these areas is vital for health. Other parts, however, such as the urine, chest, gall bladder and soft tissues, should be sterile. When these become infected (either from the patient's own body or from elsewhere), people get localized symptoms and perhaps a temperature, but usually they remain systemically well for hours or days, even without antibiotics. If the bacteria spread to the bloodstream, however, the patient can become extremely unwell. Samples of sputum, urine and even blood can be contaminated as they are collected with normal bacteria from the mouth, genitals or skin, so positive results have to be interpreted in context and with caution. However, Gram negative bacteria (a group of bacteria that stain a certain way under the microscope) aren't usually found on the skin so this result didn't fit with contamination, and when the bugs have got into your blood, particularly when they can be grown within eight hours, you are in danger. Septic shock is just round the corner and, after that, multiple organ failure.

But these were all just words to me back then, because I was still trying to work out the difference between a well patient and a sick one. They were all sick to me, that's why they were in hospital, and although I could see that some were obviously in dire straits because they were unconscious, blue, or panting like a dying soldier in a war movie, the rest were a bit of a mystery. Any one of them might drop dead at any moment as far as I could tell, and any abnormal blood result might be life threatening. I'd already rushed to my seniors like an eager six-year-old with several urine and sputum results that had grown a zoo of bacteria, only to be met with a shrug of indifference.

'Contaminant,' they'd said dismissively. 'Did you wash your hands before you took the sample?'

Maybe that was what made me feel like a six-year-old.

I had no idea what complex calculations were going on in their brains when they dished out these hilarious put-downs, so as far as I was concerned relaying Petros's result would have elicited a similarly withering response. With time to think, I might have reconsidered that conclusion, but within five minutes I'd been bleeped three more times – to take some blood, insert a urinary catheter and write up a drug chart – and soon the positive blood culture had slipped out of my mind completely, until the nurses called to tell me that Petros's systolic blood pressure was eighty.* That's low – dangerously low. Septic-shock low.

By the time I got back to Murray ward even I could tell that Petros was not doing well. He was lying in his bed with his eyes half closed, drenched in sweat and gasping.

'His pressure's dropped again, to seventy-five,' a staff nurse informed me. 'Pulse one-thirty; AF, I think.'

'Has he got IV access now?'

'No. I told you it tissued.'

Petros's intravenous cannula had dislodged from its vein, so anything we gave through it would go into the tissues of his arm

---

* Blood pressure has two components: systolic, which describes the pressure in the arteries at the peak of the heart's contraction (the pulse), and diastolic, the lower arterial pressure when the heart is relaxed and refilling (between pulses). A normal blood pressure is around 120/70 mmHg.

rather than his bloodstream. AF, or atrial fibrillation, describes an irregular heartbeat in which the smaller chambers, the atria, stop contracting effectively and all the work is left to the larger ventricles. It occurs when the heart's electrical conducting system is disrupted, either by an internal problem like a blockage of its blood supply or by an external disturbance such as sepsis, dehydration or chemical imbalance. Petros definitely had sepsis and dehydration (exacerbated by the diuretic I'd given him earlier), but we couldn't give him the fluids or antibiotics he desperately needed until he had a new intravenous cannula.

'Can you call ICU; I'm going to get a line in,' I gabbled, 'and we need some IV Augmentin and gent and a urinary catheter.'

Having assembled my kit – a cannula, a couple of alcohol skin wipes, a dressing, a 10ml syringe, a saline flush and a tourniquet – I knelt down by Petros's bed, pulled my tourniquet tight around his right biceps and started to tap different sections of his forearm to bring a vein to the surface, something that has always reminded me of stamping on the lawn as a child to encourage worms out of the ground. But Petros's forearm was pale, waxy and cold and there wasn't a vein in sight. The veins in my own arms were huge, like hosepipes that I could have cannulated with a dart from ten paces, but the only thing I could find in his was a vague sponginess in the front of his elbow. It might be a vein or it might not. This would be stab and hope.

'Sharp scratch,' I warned as I pushed my cannula through his clammy skin and then waited for a flashback of blood. He barely flinched, but I was delighted to see dark blood ooze back into the cannula hub and so I excitedly withdrew my needle and then attempted to advance the plastic cannula over it and into the vein. Immediately the plastic buckled and stuck. The blood had also stopped flowing back now and as I tried to re-advance the needle, it too stuck and then perforated the side of the buckled cannula. A purple lump was spreading under his skin before my eyes. I'd hit the vein with my needle, but then pulled it back too soon, before the outer plastic cannula was within the lumen. There was no rescuing it now, that vein was well and truly rogered.

'Shit,' I muttered as I withdrew the cannula, and then 'Fuckssake!' as an arc of blood followed it and landed on my chinos.* I could feel the sweat running down the small of my back. I pressed on the puncture site with one hand (cursing myself for forgetting to put gloves on) and belatedly released the tourniquet with the other. I'd been forcing the blood out of the vein by pressurizing the system, or, to put it another way, I'd messed up a simple cannulation about as badly as was humanly possible.

'ICU on the phone.'

'Oh, great. Can someone . . . ?' I looked around for someone who might press on the hole I'd made in Petros's arm, but everyone was busy or ignoring me, so I let go, grabbed a piece of cotton wool and tape from the drawer, applied them to the dark trickle of blood that was emerging from his elbow and placed his arm over his chest. By now there was blood on the sheets, on his gown, on the bed rail and on the floor. I was not going to be popular.

'Hi, sorry, thanks for getting back. I'm Dr Harvey's houseman. I've got a fifty-five-year-old man on Murray ward I wondered if you could come and review.'

I put my hand over the receiver and stage-whispered to the ward sister: 'Could you bleep Sophie? Sorry, tell her . . . I'm an idiot.'

'Sorry about that,' I continued into the receiver. 'Hi, yes –'

---

* Most junior doctors wear scrubs these days, but back then we all wore smartish clothes under (often grubby) long white coats, the pockets of which bulged with equipment, pieces of paper and pocket textbooks.

'Fifty-five-year-old on Murray ward,' the ICU registrar repeated back to me. 'With?'

'. . . Well, he's hypotensive, tachycardic, looks awful actually, and he's grown gram-negative bacteria in his blood.'*

'From?'

'From . . . ?' My mind was blank. Did she mean where was he from? Or where had I taken the blood from? Neither seemed very likely. These one-word questions were off putting.

'The source. Where's the bacteria coming from? Urine, bowel, chest?'

'Yes, could be his urine, he does have prostate problems.'

'Is there anything in it?'

'I'm not . . . I'll check.'

'And he's on broad-spectrum antibiotics?'

'Well, the GP had him on amoxicillin for a possible chest infection, but his chest is actually pretty clear.'

'Bloods?'

It was relentless.

'White cells are about fourteen, I think.'

'OK. CRP, temperature, renal function, urine output?'

'Umm,' I covered the receiver and called to the nearest nurse: 'Could we get set up for a urinary catheter?'

She nodded, smiled and handed me a slip of paper with some blood results.

'I've just got his biochem back, now . . . Oh.' My heart sank.

---

* I was describing shock, a state of low blood pressure and inadequate blood supply to the vital organs. Shock has a short list of causes: cardiogenic – inadequate heart pumping; septic – infection in the bloodstream causing the blood vessels to dilate and become leaky; hypovolaemic/haemorrhagic – inadequate circulating blood volume; neurogenic – damage to the nerves that maintain the tone of the blood vessels; and anaphylactic – the most severe form of allergic reaction. Petros had septic shock.

Petros's kidneys had taken a big hit and his CRP, a marker of inflammation and infection, was sky high. 'His CRP is 523.'

A normal CRP value is less than five.

'Right.'

'And his creatinine is 470.' Creatinine is a chemical cleared by the kidneys. The level in the blood should be below 100.

'Is he peeing?'

'We're just putting a catheter in now.'

'Jesus! When did he come in?'

'Just after midnight.'

'And how much fluid has he had?'

'Well, actually he had a bit of diuretic initially because we thought he might have pulmonary oedema.'

'*What?*'

'I know . . . I . . . sorry.'

The ward sister arrived at my side with a silver trolley loaded with the urinary catheter equipment and shrugged apologetically.

'Sorry,' she mouthed. 'None of us are trained to put in a male catheter.'

I'd watched one go in when I was a student and then put one in myself a couple of weeks before so I wasn't just trained, I was experienced.

'His line tissued,' I continued into the phone, 'so I'm just trying to get another one in, but he's quite tricky.'

'Have you got an SHO?'

I couldn't tell whether it was a genuine question or just sarcasm.

'Yes . . . Sophie. She's . . . coming. His potassium's only five point seven,' I added, delighted to pass on at least one piece of good news. The potassium level in the blood can rise when the kidneys fail and cause life-threatening heart problems, but usually only when it's above 6.5.

'When was that blood taken?'

'Oh . . . yeah. Few hours ago.' My good moment was over.

There was a long sigh at the other end of the phone.

'OK, I'll be there as soon as I can. In the meantime – line, fluids, antibiotics, catheter and a blood gas.'

'Thank you so much.'

'And keep a close –'

'I'm not going anywhere.'

The intensive-care registrar was matter-of-fact rather than rude, exasperated for sure and patronizing, but I didn't care. She was coming, that was all that mattered.

As I put down the phone Sophie bustled onto the ward, pink cheeked with her white coat pulled hard across her chest.

'Have you got a line in?'

I looked at her helplessly and then reluctantly shook my head. 'ICU are on their way.'

Sophie, a fizzing ball of knowledge and intent, didn't break step on her way to Petros's bedside.

'I'll get you a cannula,' I offered, and ran to the trolley to assemble the equipment. By the time I got back she'd identified her target and less than thirty seconds later had inserted a large intravenous cannula. Two minutes after that a bag of fluid was gushing into Petros's circulation, mixed in with some powerful intravenous antibiotics, and twenty-five minutes later, already looking better, he was receiving an infusion of a drug to drive up his blood pressure and on his way to intensive care.

'Can I get you a coffee?' I asked Sophie as they wheeled him away down the corridor.

'You can't sit on positive blood cultures, Jim. They kill people.'

'I know . . . sorry.'

My first visit to an ICU was the next day, when we went to see Petros on our ward round. It was a routine Nightingale-style ward,* but with half the usual number of beds and three times the amount of equipment and machines. I had no idea what anything did and I was in awe of the doctors and nurses who strode confidently from one piece of kit to the next, adjusting settings. Back then, ventilators were large boxes in battleship grey with a panel of knobs on the front. You could hear the mechanics of each breath as it was delivered and needle dials displayed the pressures and flows that were being generated. With the exception of Petros, all the patients were in medically induced comas and I found them mesmerizing. They lay in suspended animation, tethered to their beds by multiple tubes and lines, like Gulliver in Lilliput. They seemed to be marooned, their inner workings controlled by a network of machines and infusions and then displayed on a series of screens. There was probably no more equipment than there is today, less even, but like a child who remembers their primary school as huge, my memory is of overwhelming complexity. I was also struck by how precarious life was for these patients. They couldn't ring their buzzer and ask for painkillers or a bedpan. They were helpless, clinging to life and completely reliant on the skills and dedication of their clinicians.

Petros looked a different man. The drowsy, gasping, sweaty patient of the previous day was now sitting up sipping a cup of tea and reading a newspaper. It was remarkable, but I felt very much 'in the way' again and loitered behind the rest of my team as they discussed his case with the ICU registrar. The conversation seemed to be in a foreign language, filled with terms I only

* Florence Nightingale designed the classic open wards with rows of patients facing each other and a nurses' station in the middle. They have remained popular in many hospitals to this day because the nurses can keep an eye on all the patients from their central position, but the proximity of the patients to each other does increase the risk of cross infection.

vaguely recognized, but I gathered that he now had nephrostomies draining his obstructed, infected kidneys,* that his blood pressure was improving and that although his kidneys had taken a battering he'd avoided dialysis – so far, at least. I looked guiltily at the huge bruise spreading down his right forearm.

'That your work?' he asked, catching my eye and smiling.

Though it would end up being at the heart of my career, I visited ICU only sporadically over the next eighteen months, but by the time I'd finished my year of house jobs, I had learnt a lot about how to recognize a really sick patient. I'd worked out which blood results should set off alarm bells, which clinical findings needed urgent action, which ECG changes were life-threatening and which drugs I was not yet old enough to use.

Over those months the ICU doctors – the 'intensivists' – gained a slightly mythical status in my mind, because whenever I was at my wits' end trying to work out what on earth to do next to the patient who was rapidly deteriorating in front of me, they swooped in, scooped them up and mostly saved the day. I had drugs, fluids and oxygen that might tinker with the failing physiology, but they had tubes and big complicated machines that could take over completely. They were the cavalry.

Acute events still scared me. It wasn't just the thought of missing something, as I had with Petros, it was also the fear of doing something that could make things a lot worse: the prospect of giving a drug for a heart arrhythmia that might either cure it or just make the blood pressure plummet; or inserting a chest drain that should remove fluid and help the breathing, but

* Nephrostomies are tubes that radiologists insert through the flanks into the kidneys to drain urine directly back out into bags when the normal route through the bladder is blocked.

which might puncture a lung; or giving morphine that would undoubtedly alleviate the pain, but might also slow or even stop the patient's breathing.

In my third week as a doctor, before I met Petros, there was a cardiac-arrest call in the Emergency Department. The hospital was on a sprawling site and the ED was 300 metres away from the main wards across two car parks, so by the time I arrived (having sprinted as a good, keen twenty-four-year-old house officer should) I was breathless and dishevelled. I assumed I'd take on the traditional 'house plant' role of putting in the cannula and taking bloods, but as I staggered, chest heaving, past the defibrillator, the ED registrar called out, 'That's VF. Shock him, please.'*

For a moment, nothing happened, but then I realized that everyone was staring at me. We had been shown how to use the defibrillator during induction, so I dialled up 200 Joules and took the paddles confidently from their slots.

'Everyone clear, please,' I proclaimed. 'Oxygen away. Charging!'

I checked that no one was in contact with the sides or ends of the patient's trolley, pushed the paddles into the front and side of his chest and pressed the charge button next to my right thumb. Three seconds later the defibrillator beeped, indicating that it was fully charged, so I called out 'Shocking!' and discharged my 200 Joules of electricity through the patient's heart. It was exhilarating to see his torso jolt in response, but then, rather than remain in cardiac arrest or discreetly regain a

---

* VF stands for ventricular fibrillation, which describes disordered electrical activity in the heart. The result of VF is that, rather than contract in a synchronized way, the heart quivers or 'fibrillates' ineffectively and stops pumping the blood. An electric shock (defibrillation) sometimes restores the steady flow of electricity and thus the beating of the heart.

heartbeat as I'd expected, the patient sat bolt upright. Now he and I were staring at each other, our faces eighteen inches apart, he with a wild look in his eye and me with a defibrillator paddle in each hand like boxing gloves. I don't know which of us was more terrified, but he was the first to speak.

'No more electrics, please, doctor!' he pleaded in a strong Bristolian accent.

'No no, of course not,' I mumbled as I shrank away into the shadows.

It was either the most successful defibrillation in history or we'd misread the rhythm and he'd not actually been in cardiac arrest in the first place.

These life-or-death incidents terrified me and should perhaps have pushed me away from ICU and anaesthesia as a career choice.* Both jobs demand the delivery of life-threatening interventions on a daily basis, often to perfectly well people in the case of anaesthesia. I am risk averse, so on the face of it, it makes no sense for me to have chosen these hyperacute specialities, yet I did, and I probably would again.

I have thought quite a lot about why. On the one hand, if I am honest, part of the reason was the realization there were areas of medicine that I was *not* cut out for. I knew that I didn't have the dexterity, type-A personality or unwavering self-confidence to be a surgeon, and I felt that pathology and radiology were too far removed from the front line. The alternatives were the medical specialities, GP, and psychiatry, but the

---

* ICU is a relatively young speciality and, in those days, intensivists traditionally came from an anaesthetic background, because both jobs involve looking after unconscious patients on ventilators who are trying to survive a life-threatening injury inflicted by either a terrible disease or a surgeon. Modern intensivists can come from a range of backgrounds or train only for that specific role, but still the majority are also anaesthetists.

problem with all of those was their woolliness and my impatience. Everything took too long and involved too much trial and error.

'Let's try you on a slightly higher dose for a few weeks.'

'Perhaps if you cut out dairy, it might improve.'

'It could be post-viral, or auto-immune. The truth is, we may never know.'

I couldn't handle it. I needed to see the effects of what I did in real time and to understand the nuts-and-bolts physiology of those effects. When I sat as a junior doctor in an outpatient clinic or a GP surgery, I felt overwhelmed by the patients' long-term conditions. Cleverer people than me had usually been trying to make them better for years, and I found myself thinking, 'How can I get this person out of my clinic?' It wasn't that I didn't sympathize with (most of) the patients, or want to help, and I enjoyed working out what to do when they presented with specific acute complaints, but when I was faced with a long-term, complex combination of physical and psychological symptoms my natural reaction was to feel either judgemental or helpless. I knew that wasn't fair, but their years of complicated symptoms made me feel exhausted, like a teenager being dragged around a museum.

On the other hand, I liked what I saw of anaesthetists and intensivists. I liked their bottom-up, logical approach to human physiology and their ability to alter that physiology, often dramatically, with powerful drugs and machines. There were no lengthy dropdown lists of possible causes for vague chronic symptoms, it was all there in front of me. It could be complex and scary, but it made sense, and I could see with my own eyes the effects of my interventions. It also meant no clinics. This was the career for me.

Whenever I went to ICU, the consultants were there on the shop floor. They seemed to exude complete certainty, competence and knowledge – intensive care Jedi, all-knowing and all-powerful masters of their domain. If they decided that treatment had become futile, then it had. If they couldn't save a patient, that patient was unsavable. But they weren't arrogant. They wore their power lightly, with humility and compassion, and I decided that I had found a tribe I wanted to join. So I got myself onto an anaesthetic training programme, passed my exams, added in ICU training, passed those exams, and finally applied for and was appointed to my dream consultant job at University College Hospital (UCH) in London. But I never achieved that Zen-like state of complete certainty, competence and knowledge. In fact, the more I learnt, the more questions I had. I'd expected triumph and tragedy, excitement and frustration, and I've had plenty of that, but I hadn't realized how confusing it would be and how much it would change me and my view of life.

Ironically, having been attracted to the logic and clarity initially, it's now the grey areas of the speciality that I find most interesting and rewarding. I am still anxious about making mistakes (as will become clear), but these days I relish the complex ethical, emotional and human aspects of the job and I love wrestling with the unanswerable questions it poses. Rather than feel threatened, I now enjoy having my opinions and prejudices challenged, because the more I learn and the longer I work in ICU, the less sure I am about almost every aspect of it. Every day I am surprised, confused or shocked by something that happens on the unit. Often I go home still pondering an ethical dilemma, an interaction, a clinical conundrum or a 'what if'.

So it turns out that I am not a heartless psychopath who can't be bothered with people who have complicated nuanced problems. I don't need things to be clear-cut, I just need people to be at death's door, or at least critically sick, for my most inquiring and compassionate self to be revealed.

And, twenty-five years on, I still debate regularly with my colleagues about the fundamentals of the job. What is ICU for? What can it do? What should it do? And who should decide?

I don't have all the answers, but through the cases in this book I will investigate these and many more questions. And I'll tell you what happened to me and what I think I've learnt – so far.

2. The Unit

You can't just walk in. You need a swipe card, or to be buzzed through, although that seems a bit unnecessary because no one without a pass wants to be there. People only come to the Intensive Care Unit when they have to, when they're clinging to life or visiting a loved one who is. Otherwise, they stay well away. We're all glad that it exists but most of us don't want to know more than we learn from TV dramas – until we have to.

Once through the front door you're into a low-ceilinged, horseshoe-shaped corridor. Every fifteen metres in each direction is another swipe-card-operated fire door, dividing the unit into isolated sections, like airlocks in a submarine. The corridor is broad but cluttered with people and equipment – a visiting medical team trying to locate their patient, an X-ray machine, some anxious relatives hovering in hope of an update, a spare ventilator, a comatose patient on the way to the CT scanner. This corridor is the high street, the main artery; everything feeds into it. The inside edge of the horseshoe is where you'll find the lifts and staircases, storage rooms, toilets and 'plant' – a mysterious set of locked, bare breeze-block chambers that contain metal boxes, piping and ladders that disappear into darkness. Along the outside edge are the people: the patients, their relatives and the staff.

Opposite the front door, halfway down one limb of the horseshoe, is reception. It is so much more than a reception. A four-metre-square alcove, it divides the clinical side of the unit into two sections (imaginatively named North and South after a lengthy brainstorming session) and is the engine room of the

ICU. During office hours there is a receptionist at the front desk who undertakes administrative work, but behind there's a hive of other activity that continues twenty-four hours a day, seven days a week. It doubles as the junior doctors' office, the cloakroom, a second coffee room and a meeting room as well as a refuge for clinicians when it all gets too much and they need to take stock and eat chocolate (although officially food and drink are not allowed). Junior doctors squeeze together along an L-shaped desk and tap away at computer terminals, writing up notes, ordering tests and prescribing drugs while stealing each other's snacks, spreading the latest gossip and seeking second opinions.

'What do you think of this chest X-ray?'

'Do you know if we can get an MRI at the weekend?'

'Yup, the three of them, on the operating table. It had to be deep cleaned.'

Visiting teams of ologists – cardiologists, nephrologists, haematologists, etc. – pop in and perch against the filing cabinet to discuss the progress of their sickest patients. Nurses lean through the door to ask for prescriptions. Nursing assistants pack blood bottles in padded pods and send them off through the vacuum chute to the laboratories. Consultant intensivists loll in swivel chairs, catching up with the state of play and contemplating their next moves.

Turn left and you're into North, the first fifteen beds – ten side rooms and a five-bedded bay – Bay 1. Turn right and (provided you've got a swipe card) you go through the double doors into South, Beds 17 to 36 – split into three five-bedded bays, a four-bedded bay and the isolation room – Bed 32.

There's no Bed 13.

Despite a dismal view of the eternal traffic jam on the Euston Road, patients often request a single side room for privacy, but they shouldn't feel pleased to get one. They're not for private patients or VIPs (although we did keep one once for the Queen, and John Prescott got one for everyone's safety), rather they're used to protect particularly vulnerable patients and to isolate those with nasty infections. Clean and bright, if a little cramped, their walls and ceilings are decorated with large pastel spots and swirls, reminiscent of a lava lamp. (They're supposed to reduce anxiety, but when combined with weeks of sleep deprivation and mind-bending narcotics, I sometimes wonder.) The rooms are also far from private. The doors have slatted shutters that are constantly being flicked open by physios waiting to start therapy, nurses looking for the drug keys and doctors looking for each other.

The five-bedded bays are gloomy and low-ceilinged. The outsides of the sealed windows are coated with inner-city grime and the third-floor location puts them below the London skyline. Although everything inside is spotless, three thick pillars and purple paper curtains that mark the boundaries between the bed-spaces divide the bays into dark corners, even when the curtains are drawn back. After a couple of hours in a bay I crave natural light, but the staff do their best to create a calm, reassuring atmosphere. The curtains absorb a lot of sound and the nurses work quietly and efficiently, so the noises that do cut through, a metal bin lid slamming, a dropped oxygen cylinder or the beeping of an insistent alarm, jar. The patients' equilibrium is fragile, and once gone it is hard to restore. The noisy bins are cited in a surprisingly high proportion of complaints.

Each bed-space is its own self-contained ICU, independently capable of sustaining a human life. The permanent equipment hangs from the ceiling on two thick articulated gantries either side of the patient's head. They emerge from the ceiling tiles like huge white robotic arms, their arteries and veins the cables that deliver oxygen, air, suction and electricity. Standing proudly forward from the left gantry is the touch-screen ventilator – the frontman of ICU technology. It has been designed to resemble an iPad and displays graphic and numerical parameters in different colours. Even when the alarms sound the tone is resonant and reassuring, although the numbers and the actual patient often tell a different story. The monitor is mounted high behind the ventilator with its familiar display of multicoloured wiggly lines. The ECG trace is always at the top in green, blood pressure next in red (displayed in real time as a waveform from a line in the radial artery), then the venous pressure line in white, the oxygen saturations in blue, and finally, at the bottom, the level of carbon dioxide expired each breath, in yellow. I don't know why they are these colours. To label the oxygen saturation in blue when that is the colour of blood with dangerously low oxygen levels seems particularly pessimistic to me. A nice bright crimson would give a much more positive message, but the order and colours are now ingrained in my consciousness, and when people reprogram the display it upsets me. I expect to see these lines, in those colours and in that order, chasing each other across the screen towards their numerical displays on the far-right-hand side. It's the pattern I am used to and from it my brain forms an impression of the patient's condition in milliseconds, before I am even aware of it.

Below the monitor, on a small precarious shelf and hanging off the gantry in bags, are a tangle of tubes, cables, pots, canisters and plastic – suction catheters, ventilator tubing, filters, connectors, spare oxygen circuits, face masks, banks of syringe drivers and their curly delivery lines, oxygen ports, power cables and nebulizers. It is order and chaos combined. The syringe drivers and the ventilator deliver precise, carefully considered support that is constantly tweaked to match the patient's changing needs, but the sheer volume and intricacy of plastic and lines, combined with the unpredictable bodily functions of a critically sick human at the end of it, create unavoidable disorder. Reconciling the two, while still maintaining patient safety (not to mention sanity) is just another thing that ICU nurses do every day.

We used to have a huge sheet of paper, two metres square, at the end of every ICU bed, on which the nurses manually recorded everything. It was a landscape of the patient's last twelve hours. The undulations in blood pressure, pulse, urine output, oxygen levels and other physiological parameters were mapped out over the shift and the nurses took pride in this intricate document of their day's work. They were meticulous, using different colours for different body systems and often annotating moments to add context:

The physio's cleared her chest.

His daughter, whom he'd not seen for a year, visited.

But there is no paper any more. Nowadays a computer terminal is attached to the right-hand gantry by an awkward articulated arm that holds it too high to sit at, but too low if you stand. The keyboards are made of flat, slack rubber, which has been wiped clean so often that some of the letters are long gone. Logging on to certain terminals now requires a moment of letting go and allowing the 'force' to take control of your fingers.

Sharp-edged trolleys contain the rest of the kit: syringes, needles, swabs, towels, lines, cannulas, warming blankets, fresh sheets, sliding sheets, inco pads, gloves and aprons. Other items such as dialysis machines, echocardiograms, ultrasounds, spare breathing tubes and bronchoscopes are kept away from the bedside, either on trolleys in the corridor or in overcrowded storerooms. It's cluttered and awkward. There's always something in the way or tangled or just out of reach, and the box of size large gloves is invariably empty. Every bed-space also contains a sink with motion-sensing taps, because the fewer surfaces we touch the fewer infections we spread, but that's scant comfort for the exhausted registrar who leans back on one at 4 a.m. and gets a soaking-wet bum.

Side Room 32 has a slightly mystical status. Situated at the far south end of the unit, away from the other side rooms and nestled between two bays of surgical patients (most of whom have usually just dropped by for a night or two of support and monitoring after particularly high-risk surgery), it is our only proper isolation room. Equipped with a private bathroom and antechamber, it was constructed to accommodate highly infectious or contaminated patients, but with the exception of a few Covid cases it has never really done so. Alexander Litvinenko (the ex-KGB officer poisoned with polonium-210 – more of him later) was in Bed 9; a young man who'd caught viral haemorrhagic fever (not Ebola but similar – again more later) in West Africa was in Bed 7, even a tragic case of rabies failed to make it through the double, double doors of 32. The problem was that in each case the diagnosis came after the admission. To move them again, after they'd already contaminated one room, would only have increased the risks to everyone else. Instead, Side Room 32 has been used for a collection of different problems, most commonly for vulnerable teenagers who've had their immune systems annihilated by an attempt to cure a particularly aggressive form of leukaemia. Perhaps one day we'll get our radioactive Russian or our afflicted aid worker into the 'special' room.

If a patient is with us for a while the relatives often decorate their bed-space. There is a limit to what you can do with an ICU bed-space (the trollies and gantries only really come in one colour), but photographs of the patient and their loved ones in happier times make a difference – to the staff, if not always to the patient. Many of the occupants doze in a twilight zone and it is too easy to see them as just a puzzle or a set of problems to be dealt with by all the drugs and machinery. The photographs and personal items turn them back into human beings. They remind us that the person in front of us was not always so monitored, limited, flaccid and undignified. They were loved and loving, proud, important and independent. The pictures are often barely recognizable, even if they are recent, and that can be upsetting, but they're very much worth studying. Looking into the eyes of a proud father of the bride or at the smile of a tanned mother sipping cocktails on a tropical beach reminds us what it's all about.

Cut back across the horseshoe from reception, past the stairs and patient lifts and you'll find yourself on the unit's west limb – the patient-free zone. To your right, the staff coffee room marks the boundary between clinical and non-clinical. To the right of that is Side Room 1. To your left (through a locked door, obviously) you'll find the matron's office, the seminar room, the two relatives' rooms.

I can still remember my disappointment in 2005 when I first walked into the ICU staff coffee room at UCH. The hospital had just been built, and while much of it was state of the art and brilliantly designed, this room seemed to have been forgotten. It was a good size, with no shortage of industrial tea, coffee and milk, but the window looked inwards into the hospital atrium so there was no natural light, the decor was drab, the furniture sparse and the TV, now long gone, never worked. Back in 2005 a TV in an NHS staff area seemed important because, quaintly, we all used to watch the same screen together – catching glimpses of the tennis at Wimbledon or *X-Factor* between ward rounds. Perhaps the engineers who never answered our calls to come and fix it knew what was coming.

Originally, the two relatives' rooms (a large general one with tea and coffee for 'waiting' and a smaller one for private meetings between the doctors and families) were equally drab and bland, but a few years ago one whole wall of each was decorated in 'sunlight through a bluebell wood' wallpaper. I was cynical initially, thinking the choice was sentimental and chocolate-boxy, but I rather like it now. Perhaps I'm going soft in my old age.

The seminar room is scruffy, too small and an odd, irregular shape. Invariably it's half-filled with boxes and equipment that won't fit anywhere else (along with the odd blanket left by a night-shift doctor who popped in to get a bit of shut-eye), but it's a room that I feel strangely attached to. It's where the majority of our big discussions have taken place over the years. In here we meet our physio, pharmacist, nursing and dietician colleagues every day to talk through the patients over bags of crisps and soggy sandwiches. We argue about what to do with the most challenging patients (and relatives), debrief after the most difficult deaths, coordinate our response to the crises and crack the darkest, most despairing jokes. Like the owner of an old banger that promised more than it's ever delivered, I'd be loath to give it up.

Back at the bedside, the nurses are everything. Their twelve-and-a-half-hour shifts are often stressful and exhausting and their efforts can sometimes feel, to them, hopeless and pointless, but the patients rely on them absolutely. The nurses work together for washes and turns,* and cover each other for breaks, but the rest of the shift they spend with their own designated patient, administering drugs, adjusting the ventilator, clearing secretions from the chest, monitoring the vital signs, updating relatives, collecting and sending off samples of blood, sputum, urine and faeces and doing whatever the patients can't do themselves – which is usually everything. In one shift they carry out endless 'episodes of care', the details of living that we normally take for granted: clearing the throat, blowing the nose, scratching an

---

* ICU patients need to be turned from side to side every two to three hours to prevent pressure sores developing. Turning unstable, unconscious patients who are attached to ventilators requires both skill and strength, as I discovered during Covid, when I spent eight hours one day doing nothing else.

itch, blinking, swallowing saliva and shifting position. Each one is so mundane and repetitive that normally we barely notice doing them, but we certainly notice when we can't. Think of an itch under a plaster cast and then multiply it by a thousand. The nurses suction saliva, clean teeth, lubricate eyes and lips and do whatever they can to make their patients as comfortable as possible. That level of care and attention, delivered to a stranger with reassurance, compassion and good humour, is in my view one of the greatest things a human can do.

The other clinicians fit in around the nurses. We are all visitors at the nurse-and-patient's residence. As the consultant, I arrive with the junior doctors for a ward round twice a day, review everything and make a plan for the next twelve hours. We then pop back intermittently to enact those plans, catch up with relatives and troubleshoot. The physios treat chests by loosening up and clearing infected secretions with a variety of techniques and machines, and lead rehabilitation,* the speech therapists assess swallow safety, the psychologists diagnose and treat mood disorders, the dieticians calculate nutritional requirements, the

* While the patients are ventilated the aim is to have them awake enough to cough and help clear secretions from the lungs, but asleep enough to tolerate the breathing tube that passes down through their vocal cords into the windpipe. It's about the most unpleasant place you can have a tube, and while some patients stay calm with minimal sedation and are able to nod and shake their heads to questions, others become distressed, disorientated and agitated. Their brains are still too scrambled to wake calmly so they need more time, but the longer they're sedated the longer they stay on the ventilator, and the longer they stay on the ventilator the more complications they suffer. So, the next day we try to wake them again, and the next. If we're not able to get them off the ventilator within about two weeks we put in a tracheostomy, moving the breathing tube from the mouth to the front of the neck. It's much less painful breathing through a tracheostomy and most patients tolerate it without sedation and settle in for the days, weeks or even months it'll take for them to be weaned off the ventilator.

pharmacists check all the prescriptions and offer guidance and the ologists swing by to offer their specialist perspective. On a good day many hands make light work and on a bad day there are probably too many cooks, but there is a rhythm to it all. There is a structure that everyone understands and follows and it all runs smoothly . . . until . . . stuff happens. One moment it's calm, the patients are following their plans, the admissions are nicely spaced and there's a full complement of staff, but then two patients are suddenly impossible to ventilate, a third has started bleeding torrentially from their stomach, three staff phone in sick and three emergency admissions are vying for one bed. Within a few minutes the unit has transformed from intensive care to critical care, and the detail and nuance has been replaced by action and noise.

'Why can't we ventilate?'

'Where's the bleeding coming from?'

'Which of the referrals needs the bed first?'

'Get me a chest-drain set.'

'Get everything ready to re-tube Bed 6.'

'Call the anaesthetists to come and give us a hand, and gastro to scope the bleeder, and put out a major haemorrhage call.'

'If Mr Haines is still agitated just flatten him, make him safe for now.'

For a while it can feel as if we'll be overwhelmed, as if we'll lose control, but the staff know how to respond. The lack of predictability is part of the job and for some it's the reason they chose ICU. Adrenaline floods the veins and we coalesce as a new type of team: the ventilation gets unblocked, the bleeding is stopped, cover staff are cobbled together and patients are discharged to make room for the emergencies – all often in the nick of time. Almost always the necessary gets done, but occasionally, of course, it doesn't. The patient was bleeding too heavily, the cause of the ventilation problem was identified too late, the re-intubation failed or, rarely, the wrong call was made. Then an exciting busy shift becomes a nightmare and a tragedy. Then the reality of the job hits home. Then the unit transforms again, into a place filled with grief, anger, fear, guilt, blame and recrimination. Then a day we'd have forgotten within a week or two becomes one that we might never forget. Then we need to look after each other as well as the patients.

And in the aftermath of the emergency, whatever the outcome, it is hard to refocus on the everyday. The drama and high emotions make the patient who has been stuck on a ventilator staring mournfully into the middle distance for three weeks seem prosaic. The dramatic cases always draw focus, and shifting back down through the gears to devote time and energy to the mournful man or his delirious neighbour when our minds are still full of emergency takes a huge effort. For some patients, progress can be glacially slow, their ability to communicate limited and their outlook bleak. What they need is our time, our energy and a fastidious attention to detail, but as the doctor it's so easy to feel a strange combination of inadequacy, guilt and despondency. So the temptation is to nod, smile and move on. They're not getting worse, the team are doing all the right things, we can pick it up tomorrow; even though we know by tomorrow there'll be a new emergency. At our best we find that time and energy, and when we do it's invariably worth it.

The ICU occupies a space both at the cutting edge of medical technology and at the cusp of life and death. But while the machines can postpone dying, they can't make people better. The patients themselves have to do that. They must have the potential to progress from this 'existence' to a 'meaningful life' – except that no one has defined what that is. So the invasive, technical medicine rubs shoulders with profound ethical dilemmas, and it is these dilemmas that we the clinicians discuss, debate and argue about every day.

The discussion is usually constructive and consensus is reached, but not always. People have strong views about burden versus benefit of treatment and what constitutes a realistic chance of recovery. That's healthy – until difference of opinion becomes lack of respect. Then the team is in trouble.

But the goal remains profoundly simple. The unit can seem overwhelming, complex and intimidating – all lights, machines and beeps – but all we're trying to do is to support whichever bit of the body has stopped working until it starts up again, or until the patient can be moved somewhere for that body part to receive long-term support. That means that, despite being highly technical, ICU is also the last truly general ward in the hospital. It doesn't matter whether you've caught malaria, had a stroke or been shot, if a vital organ (or two) has stopped working you end up with us.

All of life is in ICU, but stripped back to the bare essentials. Wealth, power, status and dignity are all gone. There is no judgement, no deference, no hierarchy and no favouritism. Each patient is treated on their merits and our own prejudices and beliefs are pushed to the back of our minds. If there is a reasonable chance that the patient in front of us might return to a meaningful quality of life and they want to take that chance, then we offer it.

If only it was that simple.

3.   Risks

Compared with other doctors, anaesthetists die young. Two reviews of the *British Medical Journal*'s obituaries in 1995 and 2019 demonstrated that, while doctors' life expectancies overall were on average seventy-five and seventy-nine years respectively, anaesthetists died at sixty-six before 1995 and at seventy-five between 1997 and 2019. Sixty-six feels frighteningly young. There was no mention of intensive-care doctors in either study, but as the majority of intensivists are also anaesthetists, I am forced to assume the figures cover both. Back in 1995 radiologists lived to an enviable seventy-eight, although they seemed to have tailed off to a disappointing seventy-six in more recent times, but GPs now live well into their eighties.

Overall, doctors' life expectancy is higher than that of the rest of the population, probably because we are affluent and have traditionally tended not to smoke. Doctors (including anaesthetists and intensivists) die most commonly of cancer rather than heart disease for the same reasons. The vast majority of these deaths are due to a mixture of genetics and lifestyle and unrelated to the work we do, but something must be dragging down the life expectancy of anaesthetists and intensivists. At different moments through my career I've had some fairly strong ideas about what that something might be.

At 1 p.m. on 17 October 2000 I relaxed back into a saggy sofa in the doctors' mess of the Lister Hospital in Stevenage. I was four years into my specialist training in intensive care and anaesthetics and halfway through a six-month registrar placement (doing a mixture of the two specialities). The hospital was friendly, the work was interesting and, the commute from north London aside, I was enjoying it. A year earlier, I had passed my final postgraduate specialist examinations and I was still basking in the post-exam glow. I should have been concentrating on my career, but instead I was living a slightly chaotic life as a single man. My domestic cooking apparatus consisted of two microwaves stacked on top of each other on the kitchen floor.

The all-day operating list I had been assigned to had finished far earlier than planned, because the second patient was breathless after walking the ten yards from the waiting room to the examination cubicle. He also had a fever and a cough and was producing copious green phlegm, so I postponed him. He wasn't a picture of health at the best of times, and with the added burden of a lung full of infection the risks were too high. He could come back after a course of antibiotics and the month of healthy living that he'd promised. I would be reallocated to another theatre for the afternoon, but before declaring my availability, I decided to treat myself to some hospital fish and chips and apple sponge pudding in front of the lunchtime news.

'A passenger train has derailed outside the town of Hatfield in Hertfordshire,' the newsreader announced, as images of carriages strewn across an area of track filled the screen.

'Jesus!' I spluttered through a mouth full of chips.

'That's just down the road,' the medical SHO pointed out, picking his way through an irritatingly healthy salad.

'I should go and . . .' I paused and shoved two more forkfuls of fish and chips into my mouth, 'see if . . . just in case.'

I dispatched the rest of my lunch to the bin and jogged down to the Emergency Department to see what I could do. Nothing, I suspected (and hoped), but just as I got there, someone decided that our hospital should send a team out to the scene and within a couple of minutes a surgical registrar, two

Emergency Department nurses and I found ourselves in the MAJAX (major accident) cupboard donning high-viz clothing and being issued with bulky rucksacks of equipment. From there it was straight to the back of a waiting ambulance. In the confusion I managed to put on two different-sized left wellington boots, but that discomfort was soon forgotten when I looked down at my medical pack.

'PAEDIATRICS' was written in large, black letters across the bright red canvas.

'Umm,' I began, looking hopefully at my colleagues, 'does anyone . . . want to swap?' The other three pretended not to hear me as they busied themselves with fastening seat belts, checking kit and tightening straps. I didn't blame them.

None of us had been to a train crash before. We had all dutifully completed our advanced trauma life-support training, but managing patients 'pre-hospital', in this case on the tracks of the East Coast main line, was an entirely different prospect. I did not need the added responsibility of being the designated children's doctor. I had never led a paediatric trauma resuscitation and I didn't feel that this was the ideal moment to start. Aside from the emotional aspects, the physiology of children is different. The child's weight needs estimating, fluid requirements and drug doses need recalculating, lines are often more difficult to insert and they sustain a different pattern of injuries (I suspected although I didn't know for sure). This was a nightmare.

'Calm down,' I told myself. 'Stick to ABC – airway, breathing, circulation – and you'll be fine,' but drug doses, tracheal tube sizes and weight estimates were flying around my brain.

'The weight is two times the age plus four,' I mumbled to myself. That sounded right. 'But do you add the four then multiply by two or . . . I'm picturing brackets, so that means probably . . . Shit! Hang on, a one-year-old is 10kg, so that works. Good, so endotracheal tube size is age over four plus four . . .'

'You'll be all right,' the surgeon reassured me. 'We'll work together.'

'Thanks,' I replied, but I was not convinced. I was still the one holding the paediatric rucksack.

It turned out that, by the time we arrived, at the scene there was little left for us to do. The only casualties still on site were the walking wounded and the deceased, so the nurses and surgeon went to review the minor injuries and I volunteered for the grim task of verifying the dead. As I made my way along the tracks with a policeman and a railway official, I was shocked by how big the derailed carriages were up close. Some were turned onto their sides and the twisted metal was a stark reminder of the velocity and violence of the crash.

I was completely unprepared for the scene inside the train. I knew that it was going to be upsetting, but the juxtaposition of normal everyday life and such sudden, devastating tragedy was horrifying. I can still visualize the inside of the first carriage we entered: the buffet car. A fine layer of dust covered everything, several seats had been shunted into each other, food, drinks and bags were scattered randomly and most of the windows had smashed. The closest casualty, a middle-aged man, was bent double, crushed between his seat and the table in front of him.

I had never really appreciated it before, but in hospital we are one step removed from the horror. By the time trauma victims reach us they have been assessed, resuscitated and 'packaged' into something recognizable. We get a handover from the paramedics, a story and a set of important features such as the conscious level, blood pressure etc., but at the scene of a major incident there is no handover. The first responders have no idea what they will face.

I am used to verifying the dead in hospital. It is often tragic and heartbreaking, but we have a system and we can usually manage the dying process to a degree. The patient's loved ones can sit by their side, we draw the curtains to give them privacy and we have drugs to alleviate symptoms. These people were minding their own business on a run-of-the-mill train journey, catching up with some work, sipping a latte or staring out of the window when, without warning, their lives were just ended.

As we continued up the track to the last of the four fatalities the policeman took a call on his radio. He turned away from us and began an intense conversation, then a minute later he turned back and cleared his throat.

'They're saying it might be a device.'

I looked at him blankly.

'Really, do they think that's likely?' the railway official asked.

'I don't know, it's too early, but it does raise the possibility of a second device.'

At last, the penny dropped.

'Do you mean a bomb?' I asked, trying to control the pitch of my voice.

The policeman nodded. I looked around at the devastation.

'Shall we get on with it, then?' I suggested, already making my way as quickly as my two left boots would allow towards the final victim.

There was no second bomb, or indeed first bomb – the tragedy was later shown to have been caused by metal fatigue – but for the next ten minutes, until I was away from the site and safely on my way back to Stevenage, I felt distinctly edgy.

Four years later I was doing a night shift as the senior registrar on the ICU of the Royal London Hospital. By now I had a girlfriend, Tish, but I was still living with flatmates and using the microwaves more than was healthy. Earlier in the evening we had admitted Michael, a slim (bordering on scrawny) forty-six-year-old Tanzanian with severe pneumonia. He'd just arrived in the country to visit family in London, but by the time his flight landed was breathless and feverish, so he'd brought himself straight to our Emergency Department. He had a high temperature, a fruity cough and the classic clinical and X-ray signs of pneumonia, but he was too breathless to give us much more information. Within a few hours he was gasping for air, so we anaesthetized, intubated and ventilated him.* Once I had settled Michael onto the ventilator, I swigged down a coffee and checked his blood results. His neutrophil white blood cell count was high, consistent with a bacterial infection, but his lymphocyte count (the cells associated with fighting viruses) was surprisingly low. It was two o'clock in the morning by now and I had a diagnosis, so I didn't give the low lymphocyte count much more thought. He was on the right treatment (antibiotics and fluids) and he was stable on the ventilator. Whatever was causing the low lymphocytes could wait until the morning. The only job left was to insert a line into his internal jugular vein (a central line) so that we could give him drugs to support his sagging blood pressure.

Finding the vein with my needle was straightforward because he had a long thin neck. Nowadays we would use an ultrasound probe to guide us, but back then we used anatomical landmarks and hunted for the vein by drawing back on a syringe as we

---

* Putting someone onto an ICU ventilator involves filling their lungs with as much oxygen as possible, delivering a fast but gentle anaesthetic, paralysing them, slipping a curved blade with a light or camera at the end over the tongue to show us a view of the vocal cords and then passing a breathing (endotracheal) tube through the mouth and vocal cords into the trachea (a process known as 'tubing' or 'intubation'). This tube is then connected to the ventilator, which takes over the breathing function, and an infusion of sedative is started. It is very similar to the process we use when we anaesthetize in the operating theatre, but often more hazardous because ICU patients' oxygen reserves are often low and their blood pressure unstable. Things can go wrong very quickly.

advanced the needle. When blood flowed freely into my syringe, I detached it from the needle and picked up the long floppy wire from my tray. Blood continued to drip reassuringly from the needle so I slipped my wire through it and down into the blood vessel. The plan was then to remove the needle, make a nick in the skin with a scalpel and railroad the plastic central line over the wire. Finally, I would pull out the wire and secure the line in place. Unfortunately, as I pulled the needle off the end of the wire, I stabbed it through my glove and into the index finger of my left hand.

'Shit!'

My stomach dropped.

The three diseases we worry about catching from a needle-stick injury are hepatitis B, hepatitis C and HIV. The risk of catching hepatitis B (which can cause chronic liver disease and cancer) from a positive patient would be one in three, but fortunately there is a vaccine that offers 98 to 100 per cent protection and we've all had it. The risk of catching hepatitis C is about one in fifty and HIV one in three hundred. The level of risk is also affected by the type of needle (hollow needles that have been in the patient's blood vessel are highest risk – damn!), whether you are wearing gloves (a needle-stick through a glove is much lower risk – excellent!) and, in the case of HIV, the viral load of the patient (a well-treated HIV patient with an unmeasurable viral load presents a very low risk). Hepatitis C is now curable and HIV very treatable, but back then both could be fatal. I didn't know if this patient had any of these viruses, but he was from a high-risk country and he had pneumonia and a low lymphocyte count. In my mind, which was by then turning somersaults, he definitely had HIV and probably a huge viral load. I cursed myself for not thinking of it before. I was an *idiot*. I could have worn two pairs of gloves and been especially careful. I could have brought a sharps bin to the bedside to dispose of all the needles immediately. If I'd just thought of it there is no way I would have stabbed myself. I was in full catastrophizing mode.

I inserted the line in record time, pulled out the wire,[*] secured it, ripped off my glove and squeezed blood out of my pierced finger under a cold tap.

Luckily Danny, the consultant on call that night, was still in the hospital. Danny, now one of the leading ICU researchers in the UK and a ferocious clinician, is hyperactive and relentless. No stones remain unturned on his ward rounds and every decision is made as if not only the patient's but also Danny's life depends upon it. His brain and mouth work at a frightening speed, and his rigour is unparalleled. As his trainee I found him exhausting and intimidating, because I was always convinced I'd missed something or would look foolish, but these days he is my benchmark. Most of the ICU consultants at the Royal London stayed on the unit until about 10 p.m. and then, if all was well, went home to a nice warm bed, but not Danny. If he got as far as leaving the unit (which was not a given) he would hunker down under a desk in the consultants' office for catnaps between reviewing and then re-reviewing the patients.

I gave him a call, put the kettle on and sat down in the coffee room.

'Mate,' he began in his Northern Irish drawl as he perched opposite me, 'you OK?'

'So stupid!'

'Ah, no. We've all done it.'

I doubted that he had, but I was grateful for the reassurance.

'You've squeezed the finger under a tap?'

'Uh-huh.'

---

[*] Central line wires, which are about 50cm long, have been left inside the major veins of patients and only discovered years later by chance on X-rays taken for other reasons.

'And you've had your Hep B jab?'

'Yup.'

'Great.' Danny smiled. 'They've taken a sample from him?'

'I thought we weren't allowed to –'

'Sure, we can take the sample, and hold it.'

In what feels like a perverse twist of medical ethics we are not allowed to test a patient for HIV or hepatitis B or C for our benefit, unless they have given consent. If this man had one of the viruses and I'd caught it, it would take weeks for me to sero-convert and test positive (up to a year with hepatitis C), but in the meantime, until he woke up and gave his permission, I couldn't put my mind at rest by finding out his viral status. If he stayed in a coma for two months, then I'd just have to wait – unless there was a clinical reason to test him for his own sake.

'Remind me of the story?' Danny requested.

'Forty-six-year-old, just arrived from Tanzania. We haven't got much history, but raging lobar pneumonia and low lympho-cyte count.'

'Liver function?'

'Bit off, ALT* is up and he is mildly jaundiced.'

'He needs an HIV test and a viral hepatitis screen.'

I looked at Danny uneasily.

'What?' he continued. 'He's a young man from a high-risk country with severe pneumonia, low lymphocytes and deranged liver function. HIV and viral hepatitis could be pertinent to his diagnosis.'

I nodded. He was right, of course, but most importantly he'd taken control.

'I'll sort the bloods,' he continued. 'You go straight to the Emergency Department and get yourself some PEP.'

'Thanks, Danny.'

---

* Alanine aminotransferase, an enzyme found inside liver cells.

'You'll be fine.'

PEP stands for post-exposure prophylaxis, and if taken within an hour of inoculation, offers almost complete protection against HIV infection.

It was the early hours of Saturday morning and the laboratory declined to run the patient's viral tests before Monday (no urgent indication, they argued), so I took the PEP, which inevitably gave me diarrhoea, and crossed my fingers. On Monday evening the patient's blood tests finally came back negative for all three viruses. I threw the rest of the PEP in the bin and, despite being home alone, poured myself two large gins.

'It's not VHF,' the tropical diseases registrar stated confidently.

'OK,' I replied, thinking, *What the hell is VHF?* But he didn't elaborate, so I looked down at the young man who was lying on the trolley between us. VHF or not, he was extremely unwell.

We were standing at the main entrance to the UCH ICU in early 2009. I was married by now, and Tish was six months pregnant with our twins Tom and Edie.

'Side Room 7,' the ICU nurse in charge called down the corridor. 'If that's Joseph.'

As we pushed the trolley down towards Side Room 7, the registrar told me the story.

Joseph was a previously fit twenty-four-year-old who had arrived back from Mali by air ambulance a couple of hours before. He was an engineer who'd gone out there two weeks previously as part of a charitable project to build a dam in the village of Soromba. The goal was to contain water from the rainy season, which would allow the local farmers to grow crops throughout the year.

A week previously he'd developed a fever and then sweats and rigors (shivering, but with a high temperature). The local doctors felt it was probably malaria, but Joseph thought that was unlikely because he hadn't to his knowledge been bitten. Either way he was sick enough to be admitted to the local clinic, where he was treated for malaria. He was keen to stay in Mali, recover and then return to the project, but over the next few days he deteriorated with ongoing fevers and then kidney damage and everyone agreed that he needed to go home. By the time he landed at Stansted he was critically sick, so he came straight to the UCH Emergency Department and then an hour later up to the ICU. I had not taken the referral, so the first I knew of him was when the tropical diseases registrar wheeled him through our front door. His breathing was rapid and shallow, his skin pale and sweaty and he was barely conscious.

'Thick and thin film's negative for malaria,' the registrar added, 'but we're sending a PCR.' The thick and thin film meant that they had looked at smears of Joseph's blood under the microscope and seen no malaria parasites, but the parasite count can fluctuate, so it did not completely rule out the diagnosis. The PCR was a more definitive test.

Then it came to me, VHF – viral haemorrhagic fever, of course.

'And it's definitely not VHF?'

'Wrong country,' the registrar confirmed.

'Joseph,' I said, shaking his shoulder as a staff nurse attached a blood-pressure cuff. Joseph did not respond, so I pressed my knuckles hard into his chest. This time he grunted, but he didn't try to stop me.

'Blood pressure is seventy over forty,' the nurse informed us as I pushed my fingers into the side of Joseph's neck to feel for his carotid pulse. He was hot and his pulse was fast, thready and irregular.

'He's profoundly shocked,' I said, stating the obvious. 'Must be sepsis from somewhere. Pour in the fluids and let's get a tube in before he arrests.'

The term viral haemorrhagic fever describes a collection of diseases that includes Ebola, Lassa fever and Marburg, all of which can cause fevers, organ failure and bleeding. They are highly contagious, for most there is no specific treatment and they carry a high mortality. Unsurprisingly, they strike fear into many health-care professionals.

The West African Ebola epidemic was still four years away and the VHF that our tropical diseases doctors had been worried about was Lassa fever, a less fatal and contagious virus, but none the less frightening. Rather than occurring in outbreaks like Ebola, Lassa is endemic in the affected countries, constantly present with an annual attrition rate. Humans usually become infected by eating food contaminated with the urine or faeces of infected rats. It can then be passed from human to human, but none of that mattered because the tropical diseases team had ruled it out.

Through the morning and early afternoon we attempted to stabilize Joseph. We put him to sleep and attached him to the ventilator, we gave fluids and drugs to improve his blood pressure, we connected him to a haemofilter* to clear the acid and potassium from his blood and we gave him a combination of antibiotics and antimalarials, but despite all that he continued to decline. At about midday he started to bleed. He bled from his mouth, from his lines and from the puncture sites where we'd taken blood. The bleeding made him increasingly unstable and seven people were already in the room, squeezing in fluids, adrenaline and blood, when a student nurse pushed open the door.

'Message from the tropical diseases consultant,' he began,

* A haemofilter is the ICU equivalent of a dialysis machine that takes over the function of the kidneys when they stop working and clears waste products from the blood.

immediately attracting all of our attention. He looked down at the piece of paper in his hand. 'It might be VHF, Lassa fever, so please take appropriate precautions. There should be a result either tonight or first thing tomorrow.'

I looked around the room. There was blood everywhere: on the bed, on the machines, on the floor and on several people's arms. There were also other bodily fluids: sweat, sputum and urine. One by one, each of us washed our hands and arms, put on new gloves and aprons and continued the resuscitation.

'Too late now,' my consultant colleague Dave Brealey pointed out. He was up by Joseph's head attempting to rescue the haemo-filter line, elbow deep in Joseph's blood.

'Why have they suddenly changed their sodding minds?' someone asked, but none of us had the answer.

The student nurse reappeared at the door.

'Sorry, one other thing. It's definitely not malaria.'

'Great,' I mumbled.

Shortly after this Joseph's mother, father and brother joined us in Side Room 7. Despite us doing everything we could it seemed increasingly likely we would not succeed in turning things round, so we'd invited them to be with him.

About an hour after that Joseph died with his family around his bed. His organs could no longer respond to the support and gradually, despite our best efforts, his heart finally slowed and then stopped. We took off our aprons and gloves, offered our condolences to his family, washed our hands one more time and shuffled out of the room.

Fifteen minutes later we assembled in the seminar room with a cup of tea to debrief. It was a subdued conversation. I imag-ined myself at twenty-four. I'd still been a student, living a chaotic but carefree life, barely aware of my own mortality. I hadn't designed a dam in Mali, but I had spent some time in a rural hospital in Zimbabwe. It was an eye-opening experience, but it never crossed my mind that I might catch a life-threatening disease. I wondered if it had crossed Joseph's. I thought about his mum and dad and brothers trying to come to terms with this unimaginable tragedy. Joseph was 'super intelligent and ambitious', his mother, Julia, has told me since. He will be remembered for his 'infectious enthusiasm, kindness and willingness to help others'. The villagers around Soromba in Mali would confirm this. Their lives have been transformed by the Joseph Ewan Milthorp Barrage.

Everyone was shocked by the case, but we all agreed that we'd done everything possible. We were glad that he'd arrived in the daytime, when three consultants were on the ICU, rather than at 2 a.m., when one of us would have been rushing in from home. The tropical diseases consultant joined us halfway through the conversation and reassured us that the cause of Joseph's death was still unlikely to be Lassa Fever. There had never been a case reported from Mali – although neighbouring countries did have Lassa. Even if it was Lassa, he explained, it was far less contagious and lethal than Ebola.

I remember a creeping sense of inevitability, but I kept my mouth shut. We agreed to meet again the next day if the result came back positive.

At three o'clock in the morning my phone rang. I was on call, but this wasn't the ICU registrar to tell me about a potential admission, it was the consultant virologist. I had never been phoned by a consultant virologist at 3 a.m. before, so I knew immediately what was coming.

'Lassa fever?' I asked.

'I'm afraid so.'

'Oh God.'

At the time I knew little more about the disease than I have written above, so I sat on the bathroom floor staring at my phone. Should I google it? Would that reassure me or make me more anxious? I knew that I couldn't infect my family so I decided to leave it for now and went back to bed. After half an hour of staring at the ceiling I fell into a fitful sleep.

We reconvened at 9.15 the following morning. The tropical diseases consultant reassured us again that Lassa was a very different disease from Ebola. Ebola, he explained, spreads to health-care workers by direct contact with a patient's secretions or body fluids and carries a mortality rate of greater than 50 per cent, whereas Lassa has a mortality of around 1 per cent and is more akin to HIV in terms of contagion. To be at high risk you usually needed direct contamination with the patient's blood via a needle-stick injury. He did admit, however, that it was possible to catch it from a splash injury to the eye and from other bodily fluids, so we were told to measure our temperature daily for three weeks, just in case.

We were lucky. None of us became infected.

We were also asked to destroy any clothing that might have been contaminated, which meant that I ended up burning my late grandfather's forty-year-old brogues.

'Ridiculous!' my father proclaimed (correctly, with the benefit of hindsight), but I wasn't taking any chances. I picked them up with surgical tongs and dropped them into the hazardous waste bin to be taken to the hospital incinerator. I could afford a new pair of shoes every forty years, surely, for the sake of my health.

4. Bombs

The new University College Hospital was built, but not open. I'd accepted the offer of a consultant job a month previously and was attending my first UCH ICU consultants' meeting at 9 a.m. on 7 July 2005. Everything in the brand-new seminar room was white and spotless, but there weren't any chairs yet so we'd each brought our own from the building next door. I was due to start work there the following month and I was apprehensive. I'd worked with all my new colleagues before, but only as their trainee. Now I would be their peer, supposedly their equal, but they all spoke regularly at international conferences and wrote opinion pieces in high-impact medical journals. I was still worried about leading the morning ward round. They welcomed me warmly, though, and, following the announcement of London's successful Olympics bid the night before, puerile jokes about who should represent the unit at which Olympic sport were soon flying round the room. Ten minutes later, as the newly appointed departmental lead for ribbon gymnastics, I was starting to relax.

Then everyone's phones began to buzz and beep. The hospital had been put on high alert after reports of 'incidents' at several sites round London. Smartphones were still in their infancy and the Trust intranet system was not yet functioning, so the information coming through was patchy and contradictory. The chief executive's team messaged two colleagues, a slightly panicky ICU registrar called the consultant who was on call, and the husband of another colleague who was watching morning TV texted her. Within minutes a Major Incident had been declared and as the narrative shifted from power surges to explosions and then to the possibility of multiple bombs on Tube trains around the capital, the mood changed. There was no panic, but the jokes evaporated and soon several people were pacing around the room with furrowed brows and their phones clamped to their ears. We were lucky that so many ICU consultants were already on site and everyone quickly assumed different roles and responsibilities – except me, because I was not yet a member of staff. I still had three weeks left of my contract at the Royal London Hospital, so by 9.25 I was back on my bike, scootering east across town as fast as my 125cc engine would carry me.

The streets were chaotic. Sirens were wailing, people were rushing in different directions looking frightened and confused and the police were struggling to maintain order. Although I didn't know it at the time, I must have passed within a hundred metres of where the fourth and final bomb would explode on a bus in Tavistock Square, less than ten minutes before it detonated. Again, I was inadvertently heading towards rather than away from danger.

When I arrived at Whitechapel Road it was cordoned off fifty yards short of the hospital, so I shouted to the nearest police officer through my helmet visor.

'I need to get to the Royal London.'

'You can't.'

'I work there.'

'There's a major incident, it's closed off.'

'I know, that's why I need to get there.'

'Emergency personnel only, I'm afraid.'

'I am emergency . . .' I looked down at my scruffy Vespa. I did not look like a member of the emergency services. 'I need to get to work.'

'You'll have to wait. We've got ambulances coming through with major casualties.'

'*I know, that's why I have to get through! To look after the casualties!*'

'You a doctor?'

'Yes.'

I should have said that at the beginning.

'Sorry, Doc, through you go.'

I finally made it to resus* at the same time as the second casualty (the first was already two bays down, surrounded by a team of clinicians). She was in her early thirties and covered by a layer of dust, blood and grime. Her suit jacket was torn and dirty and the trousers were ripped to shreds, but she was fully conscious. As I entered her cubicle she pulled herself upright on the trolley, trying to get a view of her legs. She looked terrified.

Her lower limbs had taken the full force of the blast and were a mangled mess of tendons, muscle and skin. As we tilted her to transfer her from the stretcher to the trolley it became apparent that someone else's foot was embedded in her thigh; propelled deep into her own mutilated flesh. For a second, we froze, struggling to comprehend the horror of what we were looking at, and then professionalism kicked in and we slid her across. Her own left foot was gone and her right, still in its trainer, was attached only by a ragged string of tissue.

The ED consultant tried to calm and reassure her as two nurses took a set of observations. 'It's all right, we've got you. Has she had some pain relief?'

'Ten of morphine, IM.' The paramedic who'd brought her in replied.

'Thirty-three-year-old female,' he continued, 'extracted from the index carriage† at Aldgate after approximately an hour.

---

* Resus is the area of the emergency department where the most seriously ill patients are looked after, an ectopic mini ICU.
† The index carriage is the one in which the bomb detonated.

48

Initially hypotensive, but responded to fluids. GCS 14–15 ever since,* spontaneously ventilating, good bilateral air entry, O_2 sats 96 per cent on ten litres of oxygen. BP a hundred over seventy, heart rate one-twenty, severe injury to the right arm – and the legs . . .' He paused as we all looked down. There was no need to say anything more about her legs. 'Tourniquets around both thighs, she's had one point five litres of fluid.'

By now she was screaming.

'Can we have another ten milligrams of morphine IV, please?' the ED consultant requested, before turning back to the patient. 'You're OK, we're going to look after you. Can you tell me your name?'

'Martine.'

'Anaesthetist to the top end, please. And can we start the primary survey.'

As I made my way round to the head of the bed, the ED registrar verbalized his primary survey.

'Airway clear, breathing twenty-five breaths per minute, good air entry bilaterally . . .'

'Could you get an art line in?' I asked.

'My legs.' Martine tried to sit up again. Her arms flailed in front of her and she inadvertently slapped the nurse who was trying to take her blood pressure before slumping back into the trolley.

'I think we need to get her off to sleep,' I said. 'RSI with in-line stabilization.' I turned to the anaesthetic registrar who had just joined us. 'You happy doing the top end if I do drugs and cricoid?'

'Yup.'

---

* GCS – Glasgow Coma Scale – grades a patient's conscious level. The range of scores is 3 (completely unresponsive, even to pain) to 15 (awake and fully orientated).

'I'll do in-line stabilization,' an ED nurse offered.

'Thanks.'

'Arterial line is in,' another ED registrar confirmed.*

'Can you run a gas,' I requested.

'BP's ninety over fifty.'

'Pressure bag on the fluid, please, and we're going to need blood.' I could feel the adrenaline flowing as I tried to control the tone of my voice.†

The anaesthetic and intubation went smoothly, and after some more fluid and two bags of blood Martine was ready to be transferred to the operating theatre via the CT scanner – just as Danny called for help from two bays down.

---

* An arterial line, usually placed in the radial artery of the wrist, gives us a beat-to-beat waveform of the body's blood pressure. It also allows us to take blood samples for an arterial blood gas analysis, or ABG, which only takes a few minutes to perform on a machine in ED or ICU and gives the blood oxygen, carbon dioxide, pH, haemoglobin, sodium, potassium, lactate and sugar levels. It is a hugely useful test in acutely unwell patients.

† Anaesthetizing trauma victims poses three major hazards. First, they have often lost blood, so when we give the anaesthetic drugs that dilate their blood vessels and dampen their heartbeat, the blood pressure can plummet – hence the rapid fluid infusion. Second, they could have a broken neck, so moving their head around to get the breathing tube in might paralyse them. To prevent that, someone immobilizes the patient's head and neck between their hands while we intubate (in-line stabilization). Finally, their stomach might still be full of food, so we need to stop that regurgitating up to the throat and then down into the lungs (we usually starve people for six hours before anaesthetics to avoid this problem). We do that by using a 'crash induction' or RSI (rapid sequence induction) – an anaesthetic in which everything is done in quick succession (hence the title) and pressure is applied to the front of the neck to compress the oesophagus against the spine and stop the cornflakes or whatever coming back up. No one has ever proved that applying this pressure works, but it has been standard practice in the UK for as long as anyone can remember – although in France they don't bother.

'You OK to take her?' I asked the registrar, 'If I go and help Danny.'

'Yup.'

Danny is the ICU consultant who'd sorted me out when I'd stuck a needle through my thumb as a registrar ten months previously. If he was shouting for help it had to be serious.

Danny's patient, the third in, had been relatively stable so far, but was now becoming agitated and his blood pressure was dropping. He too had horribly injured legs and cuts and bruises all over his body, but we needed to understand why he had suddenly changed. Was it due to ongoing bleeding or could it be something else? Damage to the heart? A spinal cord injury? A punctured lung? Danny needed more hands to resuscitate and anaesthetize his patient, while he and the surgeon tried to work out what was happening, so I joined him and we prepared for another crash intubation.

On days like these there is an overwhelming urge to help and everyone turned up at resus, from the hospital's psychiatrists to its finance managers. To begin with, it was chaotic. The cramped seven-bedded area was swarming with more than a hundred people at one point, which meant that it was noisy, and the louder it got, the louder we all shouted in the struggle to make ourselves heard.

'Can we get a chest X-ray to Bay 3, please.'

'Can someone find out if there is a theatre prepped and ready?'

'Blood samples to go, Bay 4!'

'I need a second anaesthetist and a chest drain in Bay 5 and O-neg blood.'

Quickly, however, the lead ED consultant regained control and the numbers thinned down.

He divided the staff into teams. Each patient was allocated a surgeon, two anaesthetists, an ED doctor, a nurse, a radiographer and a runner. Once a patient had been assessed, stabilized and 'packaged' by the team they were transferred to the CT scanner if appropriate and then upstairs to an operating theatre. That patient's bed-space was then cleaned and restocked for the next casualty and their new clinical team. I remained in resus acting as a floating anaesthetist/intensivist, moving between the beds to help out as and where I was required.

The eight critically injured patients who came through resus that morning had all suffered horrific injuries to their legs, because the bombs had been placed under the seats, but they also had a collection of other problems. Some had chest trauma and were struggling to breathe, some were bleeding heavily and shocked and some had suffered serious head injuries. The initial trip to theatre was to assess the full extent of the injuries, identify and stop any bleeding, stabilize the vital systems and minimize any further damage. More definitive operations could wait for another day. Many of the victims had lost the blood supply to their hands or feet because bruising and swelling of the limbs had compressed their blood vessels. They needed fasciotomies (the cutting open and decompression of muscle compartments) or, if the limb was unsalvageable, amputation. The decision to amputate was potentially both life-saving and life-changing, so it was made jointly each time by three consultant surgeons: one vascular, one plastics and one orthopaedic.

Blast injury is divided into four categories. The primary injury is caused by the supersonic shock wave, which travels through the body and can damage the ear drums, lungs, long bones, brain, bowel and occasionally the solid organs such as the liver and kidneys. It dissipates quickly over a few metres, but can be reflected off surfaces such as walls so is particularly destructive in enclosed spaces. The secondary injury is caused by the debris carried in the post-shock wind. This usually travels much further than the shock wave itself and is often the biggest killer. Tertiary injury is that caused by the victim being thrown against a surface or having structures fall on them, and quaternary injury describes everything else, such as inhalation injury, burns or exacerbation of an underlying condition.

By 1 p.m. all the critically injured casualties had left resus, so I decided to head up to the ICU to see what I could do next. The overloaded mobile phone networks had been out of action for hours by then, and although I'd texted Tish from UCH to say that I was fine, I'd had no contact with the outside world since arriving at the Royal London. But as I made my way through the corridors towards the ICU, I caught a glimpse of a TV in a staffroom. I stopped to stare at the image of the exploded bus on the screen. Its roof had been blown clean off, and all that I could see of the top deck were the orange poles sticking up into fresh air out of the crumpled, flailing red panels of the lower deck. I didn't dare to imagine the devastation in the three Tube tunnels.

These days the Royal London Hospital in Whitechapel has two gleaming nineteen-storey towers, one of which contains a state-of-the-art, forty-two-bedded ICU, but back then the unit was in the old Victorian building just down the corridor from the room where Joseph 'The Elephant Man' Merrick lived out his final years. Its fifteen beds were crammed into every nook and cranny of a dark, low-ceilinged patchwork of rooms and bays. That day we had one spare ICU bed and three patients who could be stepped down to normal wards, so we'd need to move three more out to ICUs in other hospitals to make space for our seven bomb victims. The consultant on call picked out the three most stable and I was given the job of transferring one of them to our sister ICU at St Bartholomew's Hospital, two miles down the road.

It was odd, emerging from the hospital into bright July sunshine and a bank of news reporters and TV cameras, but I pretended not to notice them and focused (almost too) intensely on my patient.* The transfer was slow and frustrating, because of all the police and chaos on the streets, but my patient and I got through it and I dropped him off safely, handed over and made it back to the Royal London by 5 p.m. – only to be sent home. It was Thursday, but I would be starting my seven days on for the unit on Monday, so the boss thought it would be a good idea for me to get some rest.

Scootering back across town on that warm summer evening was a surreal experience. The streets and parks were filled with people wandering home from work. They seemed listless, bemused and slightly lost, their jackets slung over their shoulders and their shirt collars pulled open. It reminded me of the final scene in a disaster movie. When I got home, Tish was baking. She never bakes, but it was my birthday the next day and she needed a diversion from the news that had been unfolding since breakfast. She greeted me through clouds of flour with a huge hug. I scooped a finger of icing mix out of the bowl, poured myself a cup of tea and collapsed in front of the TV. For the next two hours I sat paralysed, staring at the screen, slowly taking in what had happened to London.

We didn't feel much like celebrating the next day, so Tish and I spent most of it sitting in the garden pondering the state of the world and eating cake. I felt as if I was treading water. I was fidgety and found it hard to relax. It was beautiful weather and I should have been enjoying a long weekend in the sunshine

---

* The BBC TV show *Trauma* was being filmed in the Royal London ED at the time and the different reactions of staff to the cameras was fascinating. Some loved being filmed and some hated it, but the most interesting group were those in the middle who claimed to be indifferent. I don't believe they were. I think secretly they liked it, but hated themselves for that and didn't want to admit it. Or perhaps that was just me.

before a busy week, but I couldn't. I just wanted to get back to work and do something useful.

But within half an hour of arriving in the hospital on Monday morning I was ready to go home again. Of our fifteen ICU beds, seven were now filled with bomb victims and their blast injuries were terrible.

Five of our patients had required leg amputations, one an arm amputation, two had spinal fractures, three had significant brain injuries, two had facial fractures and three had penetrating eye injuries (one ended up blind). All had suffered lung injuries and burst ear drums and two had significant burns. For the week after their admission, most had to return to the operating theatre every two to three days for further exploration and washout of their wounds.

My week on call was stressful for several reasons. I was prepared for it to be busy and of course it was, but some aspects of the clinical care were a complete surprise. It had taken forty-eight hours (while I was away) for all the victims to be identified, (during which time frantic relatives must have been phoning around hospitals fearing the worst), but by the time I came back on Monday, all the next of kin had been contacted. What I found difficult though was differentiating between them. I felt guilty when I muddled up who was due for what when, but looking back it shouldn't have been a surprise. I had never looked after a single bomb victim before and now I had seven of them as well as eight other critically sick patients. Each victim had multiple complex injuries with many similarities but also crucial and sometimes subtle differences. We should have had a huge board with it all recorded, but we'd not dealt with this number of critically sick and similar casualties all at once before. I was paranoid that in my confusion I'd miss something and went back to each patient's record again and again to check.

The other issue I'd been unprepared for was tissue transfer. The victims had all been in close proximity in a small enclosed space when the bombs detonated, so some (Martine being an extreme example) had other people's tissue embedded in their bodies. We had to check them all for blood-borne viruses (hepatitis and HIV), vaccinate them against hepatitis B and then risk assess and decide whether to offer post-exposure HIV prophylaxis. It was impossible to be sure who had been exposed to what, and if someone had contracted a virus it would not be detectable for months, but to my knowledge no one did. It was just another grim potential sequela of this vicious, indiscriminate attack.

The fact that I had never looked after a bomb victim before proved to be less of an issue on an individual basis than I had expected. I was unfamiliar with the patterns and clinical course of the injuries, but I could react to the changes in physiology and adjust my strategy accordingly. There were clinical conundrums – did an ongoing high temperature and raised inflammatory markers indicate there was new infection or was it just continuing inflammation from the blast? Should I push the surgeons to take this patient who had become unstable back to theatre or should I take them down for another CT scan? Should we start to thin the blood and risk more bleeding or leave it and risk blood clots in the veins and lungs? We face these dilemmas with all critically sick trauma patients, but because we were dealing with an unfamiliar mode of injury, we scrutinized our decisions particularly closely. As ever, it was mainly about fastidious attention to detail, but we did learn a few bespoke lessons – give broad antibiotic cover (and tetanus boosters) to all, don't let the surgeons close the wounds too soon, check everyone's ears and eyes, look out for more bleeding (particularly from amputations) and make sure your radiology reports are of the highest quality (ours were, of course!).

★

Martine needed bilateral above-knee amputations and a fasciotomy of her right arm on day one. The surgeons also opened her abdomen to look for another source of bleeding, because her blood pressure kept falling, but it turned out that the bleeding was all coming from her limbs. The shock wave had damaged her lungs too and that, combined with her need for regular operations, meant that we kept her asleep and ventilated for the first week, but by day seven she was improving so we lightened her sedation and weaned down the ventilatory support. To begin with she was agitated, confused and extremely distressed. She writhed in the bed and lashed out randomly, so we gave her sedatives and anxiolytics to keep her settled and safe, but gradually over a couple more days the fog began to lift. On day nine she seemed relatively calm and was breathing well so we bit the bullet, stopped the sedation and removed the breathing tube. For the next twenty-four hours she was all over the place. She'd been through unimaginable trauma, she could barely hear us and she had a cocktail of sedatives and painkillers still swilling around her system. It's no surprise that she was bombarded by vivid memories and hallucinations and that her sleep was filled with nightmares. She was paranoid about the multiple teams that were interrogating, poking and prodding her and I can still picture her moaning with anguish as she twisted and turned in her sheets. But towards the end of day ten (my last on for that week) she started to improve. Her family were keeping a vigil by her bedside and with their support and that of a psychologist a calm, lucid young woman gradually re-emerged. And she turned out to be remarkable.

Her full name was Martine Wright. She was thirty-three years old at the time and was commuting to her job as a marketing manager on 7 July 2005 when her life was changed for ever. She'd been out celebrating London's successful Olympic bid the night before, so she was a bit late out of bed and was rushing to work on the Circle line. The newspaper she was reading was full of the Olympics and she had just decided to apply for tickets when, four seats down from her, a fellow passenger's rucksack exploded. She spent the next hour and a quarter lying in that Tube carriage, trapped and bleeding but awake and in agony. She still has vivid memories of that time, including being baffled to see her own bloodstained white trainer hanging from a pole above her head. It was terrifying and terrible, but she never considered that she might die. She kept telling her 'guardian angel', a paramedic who was with her for most of that hour, to call her mum and let her know that she was OK.

Martine spent the next year in hospital, most of it in Roehampton rehabilitating, but the worst day, she says, was her first day out. She'd gone to stay at her mum's house, and she was grateful, but what she really wanted was to stand up, walk out of the front door and go home. That was when the reality really hit her: her life would never be the same again. Soon after that she made a decision. Unlike fifty-two other victims, she was alive. Compared to them she was lucky, she told herself, and she was determined to make the most of her second chance. Since 2005 she has married, had a baby, written a book, acquired her pilot's licence, become a campaigner and motivational speaker,* and in 2012 she didn't just get a ticket to the Olympics, she competed in the British Paralympic chair volleyball team. In 2016 she received an MBE for services to sport. Perhaps most impressively, she doesn't feel anger towards the bombers. She thinks about their families and knows that their actions must have originated from some deeply felt belief. She does feel anger towards the UK government, though, and has campaigned tirelessly for increased compensation for the victims.

*

* And a very good one – listen to her on Elizabeth Day's podcast *How to Fail*.

Six of the eight casualties who came through the Royal London resus that day survived. The seventh died of his injuries on day one in the operating theatre and the eighth died during my week on the unit. He was a thirty-year-old man called Lee Harris, who had been sitting with his girlfriend, Sam, on the Tube between King's Cross and Russell Square. Lee was working for 3DReid at Heathrow on Terminal 1's new lighting system at the time and wouldn't usually have taken the Tube to work, but he and Sam chose to that day because they had arranged to meet up with friends in the evening to celebrate their fourteenth anniversary and a friend's birthday. His parents described the couple as inseparable.

The emergency services discovered Lee and Sam lying next to each other on the tracks. Sam died at the scene, but despite severe injuries to his chest, spine, face, legs and brain, Lee was still alive when the rescuers arrived. He was bleeding heavily and suffered a cardiac arrest in the tunnel, another on the way to hospital and a third on the operating table. The surgeons opened his chest and abdomen and amputated his left leg above the knee to stem the bleeding and eventually, after a massive blood transfusion and a strong blood coagulant, he was stable enough to be transferred to the ICU. His brain was also bruised and swollen, so the neurosurgeons drilled a hole in his skull and inserted a 'bolt' to measure the pressure inside. We then tailored our ICU management to keep the pressure in his head down and the blood flow to his brain optimal, but on day six, despite our best efforts, the pressure in Lee's skull started to rise. His brain was still swelling from all the bruising and trauma and the more it swelled the less oxygen it received, which in turn led to even more swelling. It was a vicious circle. By the morning of 15 July the pressure in Lee's skull was as high as his blood pressure. Now no blood was flowing to his brain, so I called his parents in to explain the situation. They were utterly devastated, but they accepted that there was nothing more we could do for Lee and agreed that it was time to stop. They then requested that Lee's organs be considered for donation. Offering the organs of your thirty-year-old son who is dying as the result of a terrorist attack is about as selfless and generous as it gets, but Lee's parents didn't hesitate. They had no doubt that it is what he would have wanted. His kidneys were successfully transplanted and then Lee and Sam were buried next to each other in her home town of Ledbury.

Lee had thrived at 3DReid (he was described as instrumental in winning the contract for designing the Three Quays building next to the Tower of London) and his former employer now offers a bursary each year in his name – 'to continue his legacy and help new talent to find their feet'.

Five years later I gave evidence to the formal inquest into the London bombings and afterwards Lee's mother hugged me.

'Thank you,' she said. 'Now I really know that you all did everything you could and I can stop worrying that I should have fought harder for him.'

Between 9.40 a.m. and 12.30 p.m. as well as the eight critically sick victims, another 196 bomb-blast casualties attended the Emergency Department of the Royal London Hospital (most brought in on double-decker buses that had been repurposed as ambulances) and twenty-seven were admitted. By 1.30 p.m. the ED was open for business again and the next day elective operating resumed. There was no time to pause and reflect. The Royal London is a busy trauma teaching hospital and the city's traffic accidents, stabbings, heart attacks and cancers weren't going to wait for us to take stock and gather our thoughts.

None of this seemed odd to me at the time. It was a shock to be in a city that was under attack (particularly when there was another attempted bombing two weeks later and one of the bombers was chased through UCH), but work wise I think we all just got on with it. Everyone dropped everything, petty differences were forgotten and the whole team focused on one thing – the victims. As we'd see again fifteen years later when Covid-19 struck, the crisis brought out the best in us and in the NHS in general. There was a risk that the bomb victims would draw all the attention and that the other patients would get a second-class service, but with the help of our neighbouring hospitals I think we were careful to avoid that too.

I was thirty-five at the time and nervous about what lay ahead of me as a consultant at UCH, but in the cramped Royal London ICU I felt confident. I'd seen a lot of trauma over the previous year and so, although I'd never experienced anything like the 7/7 bombings at the time, I took it in my stride. I felt desperately sad for the victims and their families, but I don't remember having flashbacks or ruminating in the weeks and months that followed (as I would later with Covid). When I looked back years later it seemed odd that I'd witnessed such horror and moved on with relative ease. Perhaps it was my time of life and the fact that within three weeks I'd started on the next stage of my career at UCH. Over the years, though, I've thought often about that day and the subsequent week. I've followed Martine's career with nothing short of awe, and whenever she achieves another inspiring milestone I think back to that young woman waking up in the ICU after such horrific trauma.

About ten days after the 7/7 bombs the Queen visited the Royal London Hospital and we were asked if we would like to meet her. The ICU doctors and nurses hung back bashfully, but luckily six surgeons stepped forward to offer their services immediately.

5. Poison

In November 2006 I had been a consultant at UCH for fifteen months. My working pattern, which would change little over the next fifteen years, except during Covid, was to do a busy seven-day stint on the ICU (including three or four nights on call) followed by three lighter weeks of anaesthetics and non-clinical activities (teaching, supervising trainees, recruitment, audit, chairing meetings and the odd trip to lecture at a conference). I was growing into the job and starting to enjoy my ICU weeks as well as the Fitzrovia location, but I was still intimidated by my consultant colleagues. On Sunday 19 November I took the handover of the South half of the ICU from Paul, a fellow consultant and clinical director of acute services. Paul is one of the most effective people I've ever met. Within a year he'd be running half the hospital and four years after that directing a hugely successful private medical business. He doesn't mess about and the handover was succinct and to the point, but everything seemed under control, until at the end of the call he added as an afterthought, 'Oh, John's got the Russian spy, by the way.'

John, another consultant, would be looking after the North half of the ICU for the week, but I had no idea what Paul meant by 'the Russian spy'. I had been out of touch on holiday for ten days, but his tone suggested that I should know, so I didn't ask.

'Right, good. Thanks, Paul. I'll see you soon.'

I hung up and logged straight on to the BBC website.

When I arrived at the hospital the next morning, the first thing I noticed was a collection of vans, satellite dishes and journalists camped on the central reservation of the Euston Road. The security guards at the main entrance seemed a bit twitchy and up on the unit there was a buzz of nervous energy. Alexander Litvinenko was occupying Side Room 9 and the police had taken over Side Room 10.

The morning handover took a little longer than usual because the inevitable remarks about James Bond and ricin-tipped umbrellas slowed things down, but for most of the day, apart from seeing John disappear into rooms for meetings with various serious-looking people, I had no more to do with Litvinenko. I was the consultant on call that night, however, so I joined John for his afternoon ward round and before we entered Side Room 9 he told me the story.

Litvinenko had developed abdominal pain along with vomiting and diarrhoea on the evening of 1 November. At his request, his wife called an ambulance at 3 a.m. on 2 November but, having assessed him, the paramedics diagnosed gastroenteritis and suggested he stay home and keep hydrated. Over the next thirty-six hours, however, his symptoms worsened, so on 3 November she called an ambulance again, and this time he was taken into Barnet General Hospital. By then he was significantly dehydrated, the pain was more severe and the top of his abdomen was tender to the touch, so the Emergency Department doctors collected a stool sample and sent off some blood tests. The blood showed a high haemoglobin count consistent with dehydration, a high white blood cell count and C-reactive protein (CRP) consistent with infection or inflammation, and impaired kidney function, which again would fit with dehydration and mild jaundice. The doctors admitted him for intravenous fluids, pain relief and, in case this was salmonella or a similar bacterium, antibiotics.

Over the next few days Litvinenko (at this stage going under the pseudonym Edwin Carter) started to feel better. The diarrhoea continued, but his haemoglobin and white blood cell count settled and by 7 November he seemed well enough to be discharged home. His blood tests, however, told a different story. Now his white blood cell count was abnormally low and his platelets (the blood cells involved in clotting) were also on a downward trend. That day his stool came back positive, but not for salmonella, for the bacterium *Clostridium difficile*. *C. diff.* is a common cause of diarrhoea within hospitals, but rare in a well young man from the community.

When the doctors told him about the *C. diff.*, Litvinenko changed his story.

He explained that his name was actually Alexander Litvinenko (he never really sounded like an Edwin Carter, to be honest), and that he had been an agent of the FSB (the Russian Federal Security Service or Federal'naya Sluzhba Bezopasnosti, successor of the KGB), but had had to flee Russia because he faced a lengthy jail sentence after exposing government and security-service corruption. 'I am an enemy of the Russian State and I know that the FSB use *C. diff.* as a poison,' he informed them in his thick Russian accent.

Later I discovered that, on the day that he became ill, Litvinenko had been busy. First he'd met an Italian politician, Mario Scaramella, at the Itsu sushi bar in Piccadilly to discuss, among other things, the recent murder of the Russian journalist Anna Politkovskaya. Both men suspected that the murder was a government-sponsored assassination and Scaramella brought papers relating to an alleged Russian hit list. The documents suggested that Scaramella and Litvinenko's names were also on that list.

Litvinenko then went to the Millennium Hotel in Mayfair for a tea-time business meeting with two former FSB colleagues, Andrei Lugovoy and Dmitri Kovtun. There he drank the now infamous cup of herbal tea, while his erstwhile colleagues drank lager in preparation for an evening watching Arsenal at their new Emirates stadium and then, finally, Litvinenko continued on to the office of his boss, the exiled Russian oligarch Boris Berezovsky, to make copies of Scaramella's papers.

Usually when I tell people they've got a C. diff. infection, they either stare at me blankly because they've never heard of it, or react with a combination of worry and anger because of its reputation as a dangerous hospital superbug. No one has ever cited it as evidence of state-sponsored poisoning, but the doctors didn't doubt Litvinenko's knowledge or sincerity. The C. diff. did not explain his falling blood counts, however, so the hunt for a unifying diagnosis continued.

For the next few days, he felt reasonably well, but his white blood cells and platelets fell to dangerously low levels, leaving him at risk of infection and bleeding, and on 13 November his hair began to fall out. Next he developed a fever and the lining of his mouth and stomach became inflamed. He looked like someone who was receiving powerful chemotherapy – something was destroying all the rapidly dividing cells in his body.

The team at Barnet undertook extensive investigations, including examination of his bone marrow and a full viral and heavy-metal screen. They even passed a Geiger counter over him to check that he wasn't emitting radiation and he wasn't – at least, not gamma radiation.

Eventually something came back positive. His urine thallium level was 30mmol/L, three times the upper limit of normal. I had no idea what that meant, if indeed it meant anything, but it was a positive result so, understandably, everyone leapt on it. Stories circulated widely in the press that thallium (or even radioactive thallium) poisoning was the diagnosis. The treatment was Prussian blue (a chemical suspension that he described as 'like drinking shards of glass'), which would bind any Thallium that was still within his guts and stop it being absorbed into his system, intravenous nutrition, antibiotics, platelets to reduce the risk of bleeding, a drug to stimulate white blood cell production and pain relief.

On 17 November Litvinenko was transferred from Barnet Hospital to UCH, because we are the regional haematology centre and his low blood counts were now a major problem. He was still vomiting and losing weight, and his heart was starting to show signs of strain on the ECG, but he was awake and his vital signs remained stable.

At UCH we also repeated his urine thallium level test, and this time it came back as less than 10mmol/L – normal. His presentation did not really fit with thallium poisoning, because he had none of the neurological signs, but it was the only positive result we'd had. Now we were back to square one.

An unexplained illness of natural causes was the front-runner, but the Health Protection Agency (HPA)* was also considering deliberate poisoning with an alkylating agent such as melphalan or a mustard derivative, as well as external beam radiation. Apparently, one technique is to remove the target's car door and replace it with an identical but radioactive one. The HPA felt that internal radiation poisoning was extremely unlikely.

On 19 November Litvinenko's ECG started to look abnormal and his pain was increasing, so they moved him down to the ICU for closer monitoring.

When John and I arrived at Bed 9 the next evening there was a lot of activity, but most of it was non-medical. Litvinenko had given several interviews through the day, not just to the police but also to trusted friends and associates. These were to be released to the press alongside the famous photograph of him

---

* The HPA was a public body set up by the government in 2003 to protect the public from infectious diseases and other environmental hazards. It was dissolved in 2013 and replaced with Public Health England.

lying in his ICU bed, bald and pale but defiant. He was convinced that he had been poisoned by the Russian state and he was determined to tell his story.

I introduced myself and asked how he was.

'OK,' he replied, quietly.

'Is the pain under control?' John asked.

'Not too bad.' He rubbed his upper abdomen.

The conversation continued for a few more minutes. We checked with his nurse that there were no other concerns and then we moved on. There was no more to say. He was stable, stoical and focused.

'Thank you,' he said simply as we left.

The next day Litvinenko deteriorated. He had a fever despite antibiotics and his kidneys began to fail, causing his blood to become acidic. John treated him with fluids and sodium bicarbonate to neutralize the acid, but the following evening (22 November) he developed a florid rash, he became hypothermic and his blood pressure dropped. Now his heart was failing and, despite efforts to support it, at 11 p.m. he vomited, collapsed and suffered a cardiac arrest. He was successfully resuscitated, but his heart stopped again just before 1 a.m. John was on call that night and resuscitated him for a second time. He and the team searched for a reversible cause of the cardiac arrest,* but apart from a general decline in the strength of his heartbeat there was nothing obvious, so they put him on the ventilator, began artificial

---

* There are eight reversible causes of cardiac arrest, the four H's: hypoxia, hypovolaemia (lack of fluid in the circulation), hypothermia and hyper/ hypokalaemia (high or low potassium levels in the blood) and the 4 T's: thromboembolism (a big blood clot in the lungs or heart), tamponade (fluid build-up around the heart), toxins (you name it) and tension pneumothorax (air trapped outside the lung that compresses the heart and lungs). If the heart still doesn't beat when all of these have been corrected then there is no more we can do.

kidney support and infusions of drugs to drive his heart and push up the blood pressure and suctioned the residual vomit from his lungs.

I later discovered that on 22 November gamma spectrometry of Litvinenko's urine had revealed a trace of polonium-210. This was most likely to be a red herring, the experts from HPA thought, because there are traces of polonium in the environment, including in cigarettes, but the diagnosis of polonium poisoning still needed to be excluded. Polonium-210 predominantly emits alpha radiation, so the nurses dutifully collected a twenty-four-hour urine sample and sent it off to the Defence Science and Technology Laboratory at Porton Down for alpha spectrometry.

Over the next sixteen hours Litvinenko remained critically sick and unstable. His heartbeat became irregular and the support for his blood pressure steadily increased. I was on call again on the Thursday (23 November), and at about 6.30 in the evening, not long after the ward round, a small, late-middle-aged woman who put me in mind of Miss Marple arrived on the unit. She told me that she was from the Health Protection Agency and that she'd be grateful if we could lend her an office with a telephone. She had work to do, she said, and was waiting to receive some important information.

'Sure,' I replied, with the plots of several spy novels swirling around my brain. 'You can use the hot-desk office.'

I showed her into the narrow room, pushed aside a Brompton bicycle and picked up three dirty coffee mugs.

'Would you like a cup of tea?'

'No, thank you. I am fine.' She held up a thermos, smiled warmly and then waited. 'I will speak to you later.'

'OK, great. Thanks.'

I took the hint and left her to it.

Shortly before 9 p.m. on 23 November 2006 Alexander

Litvinenko suffered a third cardiac arrest. This time, unsurprisingly, despite nearly an hour of resuscitation and an exhaustive search for a reversible cause, we could not bring him back. Eventually, in the presence of his father, we accepted the inevitable and terminated CPR.

I emerged from Side Room 9 at 10 p.m., somewhat shell-shocked. I had been a consultant for a little over a year and this man was the lead item on the national news. He had died on my watch and I didn't know why. Had I missed something, and in doing so failed to avert an international diplomatic incident? But before I could think any more about any of this, I needed to talk to Litvinenko's wife, Marina, and their twelve-year-old son, Anatoly, who had just arrived on the unit. They'd been called in during the cardiac arrest and were waiting for me in the small relatives' room. I think they already knew that he'd died, but I couldn't be sure so I sat down opposite them and introduced myself.

'I am so sorry,' I continued slowly, 'but I am afraid that Alexander suffered a further cardiac arrest this evening and this time despite nearly an hour of CPR we could not bring him back. I'm sorry.'

I don't remember exactly what Marina said, but I do remember that she thanked us for everything and that both she and Anatoly were incredibly calm.

I asked if there was anything else I could do, but there wasn't, so I left them in the capable hands of one of our senior nurses and went back to the unit to work out what needed to be done next.

Half an hour after that, I read out a statement to the press. As I made my way across Euston Road one of the journalists asked who I was. I flashed my hospital badge and explained that I was the ICU consultant on call, but that seemed to confuse him, so I clarified.

'Intensive Care Unit.'

He still looked far from convinced, but we were standing in the middle of the road so I smiled and continued on my way.

The hospital communication department had written the statement that I was to deliver and then the police had redacted certain sections so the text jumped randomly across the page. That is my excuse, anyway, for the awkward, barely audible performance that appeared on Sky News later that night above the words 'Jim Down, Hospital Spokesperson'.

Sometime during the next hour, Miss Marple reappeared and asked if she could have a word.

'We know what killed him,' she confirmed as I shut the office door behind us. 'Radioactive polonium-210.'

I stared at her. I had not been privy to the previous discussions about the outside chance of polonium poisoning. I had never even heard of it. She might as well have said he'd been killed by kryptonite.

'Does that mean we could have . . . done something?'

'Massive dose. He didn't stand a chance.'

'Wow! Urm, right.'

I tried to hide my shock and bewilderment.

'And it's a secret. You mustn't tell anyone, until we have more information,' she concluded.

'What about the staff?'

'No one. Too sensitive.'

'But they've been in contact with him . . . isn't there a risk they –?'

'They should be fine, as long as they wore universal precautions. Polonium emits alpha radiation, which can't penetrate a piece of paper, let alone human skin. He must have ingested it somehow, swallowed it or inhaled it.'

My head was swimming. Universal precautions meant a flimsy plastic apron that often disintegrates as you take it off the roll and, for certain tasks, a pair of gloves. Litvinenko had suffered three cardiac arrests. Resuscitation is chaotic and messy, so multiple members of staff had come into contact with his body fluids. He had vomited into the face of the doctor who'd put the breathing tube down into his lungs. Would that vomit have contained polonium? And, if so, how much? And how much was too much? The nurses had handled his urine, sweat and blood. Could we be sure that they'd not been put at risk? If they had, they had a right to know.

The difficulty was that not only had I been instructed not to tell anyone, I also didn't know enough to give people useful information. Having never heard of polonium-210, I obviously knew nothing about its radioactivity or distribution through the various body fluids. And what did she mean by a massive dose? Even if she'd told me in becquerels or sieverts or curies I would have been none the wiser. I tried to visualize the periodic table in the hope that polonium might jump out at me, but I couldn't even remember the positions of the elements I had heard of, let alone this new one. I knew that half-baked information would probably only increase anxiety and I was still intimidated by this soft-spoken, polite, but steely woman who had spent the last four hours drinking her own tea and making telephone calls in our office. I did not want to get on the wrong side of the police or the secret service or Vladimir Putin, so I decided to tell just one person. My boss, Geoff Bellingan, then clinical director of ICU and now medical director of the hospital, is usually unflappable. He has seen it all before, but the news about radioactive polonium was met with silence at the other end of the line.

'I'm sorry to bother you,' I added lamely, 'but I've been told it's a secret.'

'So, you rang me.'

I paused.

'Our secret.'

'Thanks.'

Looking back, it's possible that Geoff's reaction related in part to the fact that just forty-eight hours earlier he had made a statement to the world's media explaining confidently that radiation poisoning was very unlikely to be the cause of Mr Litvinenko's illness. His words live on in the archives of *Private Eye*. We agreed that, on balance, the risk to staff was probably low and that telling them that night would be of little benefit and so we decided, as instructed, to wait until the morning.

The police then sealed off Side Room 9 as a crime scene – for two days. Litvinenko, along with many valuable pieces of ICU equipment, remained inside, while the police rushed around London frantically testing for radioactivity in all the places he had visited on 1 November. Finally, on 26 November, two men in full hazmat suits with respirators arrived to examine his room. This was years before Covid and I had never seen anyone wearing this type of protective clothing in real life. It reminded me of the famous scene in *E.T.* when the alien and Elliot become sick together (as a child I found the alien creepy and wanted Elliot to get as far away from him as possible, but I gather that wasn't the reaction Spielberg was going for). An hour or so later the two men emerged and informed us that their work was done and that we could move the body to the mortuary, which the porters did – in full . . . T-shirts. A few weeks later I read in a newspaper that Litvinenko's post-mortem had been one of the most dangerous ever undertaken. The pathologists wore full protective clothing and the burial was to be in a lead-lined coffin. They should have got hold of some of our thin plastic aprons or borrowed the porters' T-shirts.*

The morning after Litvinenko died the cause of death was

---

* Recently I visited Litvinenko's grave in Highgate Cemetery. His headstone is cut off at an angle to indicate a life cut short and stones sit on it, placed by people who knew him, to keep his memory alive. The guide reliably

released to the media and the atmosphere in our ICU staff room deteriorated dramatically. Immediately there was suspicion. Who had known what, when? Had staff been put at unnecessary risk? Did the bosses care more about espionage and clandestine activity than the well-being of their co-workers? The reality was that none of us had the information until after Litvinenko died, but many people didn't believe that. Rumours spread like wildfire, and with hindsight there is no doubt that we made mistakes. Many staff heard about polonium-210 from the BBC news bulletins when we should have been the ones to tell them and conversations in the coffee room could have been more sensitive and careful. Doctors talked about writing up the case and publishing it in a highbrow medical journal, while pregnant nurses were still worrying about the dangers to their unborn babies.

It took weeks to re-establish relationships and trust on the unit and I learnt a valuable lesson. My responsibility is to the health and well-being of my patients and staff. That has to be my priority. Others, such as the police, politicians and the press may have other pressures, but I need to stay focused on my duty of care.

Two days later all the staff who'd had direct contact with Litvinenko were asked by the HPA to collect a twenty-four-hour urine sample, to be checked for polonium. I don't think any of us thought we were going to die of acute radiation sickness, but we were worried about the long-term effects. Would we be at increased risk of leukaemia or other cancers or cardio-vascular disease in the future? Could the nurses' unborn babies be affected?

---

informed me that the 'lead-lined coffin' story is just an urban myth. His coffin is wooden.

Two weeks after handing in my sample I received a letter on HPA headed notepaper. It read:

Dear Dr Down,

Your polonium levels are of no concern to us.
Kind regards,
Etc., etc.

Wonderful, I thought. Phew! What a relief!

Then I re-read it.

What if it meant: 'Your polonium levels are of no concern to *us*'?

I didn't really care if they were concerned or not; what I wanted to know was whether *I* should be. They might view me as an expendable item. As long as I wasn't going to spread my radiation to other people, why should my long-term risks be their concern? This was an international incident, one junior ICU consultant was a small price to pay in the grand scheme of things.

As of 2022 I have suffered no complications of radiation poisoning. It transpired that no staff members were contaminated with toxic levels, so perhaps I was too quick to judge our flimsy aprons. And I did get my one and only (slightly guilt-edged) publication in *The Lancet*.

The episodes I've described in the last three chapters have certainly nourished my hypochondria, but do any of them pose significant risk to the lives of anaesthetists and intensivists in general? Which of these, if any, are responsible for our less than inspiring life expectancy?

Infection seems an obvious risk, but the vast majority of our patients pose no threat to us. We can pass some infections on to other vulnerable patients if we don't wash our hands, but usually the bugs only cause us problems if we are immunocompromised.

Yet most doctors and nurses have experienced that sinking feeling – as I did – when a contaminated needle pierces our skin after a procedure. We fret and kick ourselves for days, sometimes weeks or months as we wait to discover our fate. My best friend stabbed himself with a needle contaminated with hepatitis C infected blood and had to wait a year before receiving the all-clear. I think I would have descended into a spiral of bitterness and pessimism, but he seemed remarkably cool about it, and with good reason. It's extremely rare to pick up hepatitis or HIV at work. Since 1997 every significant occupational exposure (SOE) has been reportable to Public Health England, and up to 2018 there had been 8,765 reports. Over those twenty-one years, twenty-three health-care workers contracted hepatitis C (seven of whom were doctors), one caught HIV (back in 1999) and there were no cases of hepatitis B. Sharp implements will always be a part of medicine, so the risk is unlikely to be eliminated completely, but twenty-four cases in twenty-one years across the UK is a risk that I can live with, especially now that both diseases are treatable.

So if infection isn't going to get me what is?

People have argued about the adverse effects of anaesthetic gases on health-care workers for decades. When I was training we almost always put people to sleep with an intravenous drug called propofol (the medication that killed Michael Jackson, but is safe in a monitored environment in the hands of trained professionals) and then kept them asleep with inhaled gases for the duration of the operation.* At the end of the surgery we turned off the gas and the patients breathed it out and woke up.

---

* Strictly, the 'gases' are vapours, originally chloroform and ether but now much safer and less flammable alternatives.

The medical staff are potentially exposed to the same gases as the patient during procedures, so there are standards about the allowable levels in the atmosphere and we use scavenging (pipes that remove the gases from the operating theatre to be released into the atmosphere) and ventilation systems to ensure that these are not exceeded. Concerns have been raised that chronic low-level exposure may increase the rates of cancer, liver and kidney injury, birth defects and miscarriage, but a large study in 2016 found no conclusive evidence of harm as long as the laid-down standards were adhered to.

I have all but stopped using anaesthetic gas. I keep my patients asleep with an intravenous infusion of propofol, but not because of the risk to my own health. I have switched because it's better for the patients (less nausea, potentially improved cancer survival and a crisper wake up)* and because, once pumped out into the atmosphere, the gases exacerbate the climate catastrophe.

So why do anaesthetists and intensivists die young? Few of us are killed at the scene of a major incident, we hardly ever catch tropical diseases or blood-borne infections and radioactive Russian spies are rare. Anaesthetic gases may well be destroying the planet, but they are probably not shortening our lives, and even through the Covid pandemic our excellent PPE meant that intensive care turned out to be one of the safest places to work.

There was something else going on, but it would be a few more years before I fully appreciated what it was.

---

* There is growing evidence that the differing immune effects of various anaesthetic agents alter the chances of some cancers recurring.

6. Friends

My relationships with patients are usually short term. If they are not unconscious when I meet them, I often render them so within minutes. In the operating theatre I accompany that with light banter:

'What would you normally be doing on a Wednesday morning?'

'Got a treat planned for afterwards?'

'That's fentanyl I've just given you . . . Yes, it is a bit like heroin.'

In ICU the chat is more subdued and focused, but I don't really get to know the patients in either setting. I find out whether they are in pain, confused or nauseous and how they slept, but I don't get a deeper sense of the person and how the whole experience is affecting them. Some patients stay on the ICU for a few weeks, but they're rarely at their best and I didn't know them before, so my insight is limited. Were they always this reserved and taciturn or were they previously the life and soul? Sometimes I get an idea of what they were like in happier times from conversations with their families and the photographs by the bed-space, but it's never the full story.

Then two friends ended up in ICU. I saw how it changed them and I got to ask them what it was really like.

Sean is a freelance IT consultant. He is softly spoken and cautious, with a wry sense of humour and a highly developed interest in his own health. Google has not always been his friend when it comes to assessing his daily symptoms and niggles, but as a keen hypochondriac myself I sympathize with his position. Our wives were at school together and, as well as being good friends, we have an unspoken arrangement: he calls me about ailments he might or might not have and I phone him when I can't make my computer work. Until 2008 I'd definitely had the better of the deal, but that year he started to make up ground.

At the time he and his wife, Marina, had a three-month-old baby, Henrietta. They were living in a cramped flat in Islington, but had just started, blearily, to consider a move out of the city. It was to be one of those moments in life when everything seems to happen at once.

First, Sean was diagnosed with kidney stones, which required several discussions about specialists and lifestyle modifications, and then he developed a blocked and inflamed gall bladder. I put him in touch with a surgeon who recommended the removal of Sean's gall bladder (once the offending gallstone had passed and the acute attack had settled) to avoid future problems. Sean and I then embarked on a series of conversations about surgeons, anaesthetists, surgical complications, anaesthetic complications and private versus NHS care. Soon I was feeling much less guilty about my IT support calls.

A month later Sean phoned to say that he had pain in his upper abdomen.

I assumed that Sean's pain was either from his gallstones or gastritis, so I suggested he take some antacids and paracetamol and reassured him that it would settle down. Almost all of my friends had had gastritis in the previous year or two from too much beer and curry. We were at that age.

The next day, Marina called me. The pain hadn't settled down and Sean was now an inpatient at UCH. He had been in agony all night with a high temperature and vomiting and a CT scan had revealed acute severe pancreatitis.

The pancreas is a fish-shaped organ that sits behind the stomach across the top of the abdomen. It releases digestive enzymes into the intestine as well as producing the hormones insulin and glucagon that control sugar levels in the blood. The bile duct, which transports bile from the liver and gall bladder to the intestine, passes through the head of the pancreas.

In pancreatitis, the enzymes become activated while still in the pancreas, causing irritation of the cells and then inflammation. It is commonly caused by gallstones (as in Sean's case), or alcohol, but sometimes just happens for no discernible reason. Acute pancreatitis describes sudden onset of the inflammation and can be mild and self-limiting or severe, self-perpetuating and occasionally life threatening. At a certain point areas of the pancreas lose blood supply and start to break down and necrose (die), which leads to more inflammation and further enzyme leak. Fluid often builds up in pockets around the organ, which can then become infected and require drainage. The inflammation erodes structures outside the pancreas, most worryingly arteries, which might then burst, leading to catastrophic internal bleeding. Other organs, such as the lungs, kidneys and heart, can also start to fail. There is no way to stop it. The disease must run its course. All we can do is remove the driver (gallstones or alcohol), support the patient, manage the complications and wait for the body to (eventually) heal itself.

On my way to see Sean I'd spoken to his surgeon, who'd told me that the scan did not look good. Areas of Sean's pancreas were already necrotic. He had a huge battle ahead of him.

I felt nervous and guilty as I approached his bed, but Sean had had a slug of morphine and was much more comfortable. He looked grey and washed-out but he had stopped vomiting and was back to his usual understated, charming self. He even joked about my misdiagnosis. I was shifty and evasive. All I could think about were all the patients with CT scans like his who'd spent months on our ICU. I felt dishonest for not explaining what lay ahead of him, but I didn't know for sure. Perhaps he'd turn around quickly, in weeks rather than months, and, anyway, I was there as his friend, not his doctor.

It's tricky having a friend who is a patient in the hospital. The natural instinct is to try to push them to the front of every queue, get multiple opinions from all your favourite experts and micro-manage their care, but that can be counter-productive (quite apart from being unfair on everyone else). Not only does it inevitably upset the doctors and nurses who are trying to get on with their jobs, it also results in too many cooks producing conflicting messages and muddled plans. But as a patient in a large NHS hospital it is easy to feel powerless, so knowing that there is someone on the 'inside' whom you can call at any time is reassuring.

Within a week or two patients with necrotic pancreatitis have a certain look: sallow, sweaty and inert. They lie in the same position for weeks on end – the 'pancreatitis position' – slumped down the bed with their chin squashed into their chest and their distended abdomen bulging forward like the top half of a beach ball. The disease seems to diminish them both physically and mentally, leaving the impression that they have surrendered to a state of inert helplessness. It is a frustrating and sometimes depressing disease to manage. Scrupulous nursing care, physiotherapy and vigilance are the mainstays of treatment, along with support of any organ that fails, regular CT scans, antibiotics if there is an infection, nutrition and occasionally an intervention to drain a fluid collection or block off a bleeding artery. Progress can be painfully slow and I have always had huge sympathy for this group of patients, but Sean gave me a new level of insight.

He spent the next four months in UCH, the first five weeks of which were terrifying. His second CT scan looked worse. The pancreas was digesting itself and releasing toxic enzymes and chemicals into his abdomen that were starting to threaten other local organs and blood vessels. Despite having two fluid collections drained he continued to deteriorate, so we moved him down to ICU for closer monitoring and support. Now his whole body was inflamed. His temperature and heart rate were up, his blood pressure was down and his breathing getting more laboured. He was behaving like someone who had sepsis – an infection in the bloodstream – but antibiotics would make no difference to Sean, because this wasn't caused by bacteria. It was all coming from the inflammation of his pancreas.

After three weeks, Sean hit crisis point. His latest CT scan looked awful. The fluid collections were growing, despite drains; there was dead pancreas perilously close to fragile arteries and the lungs and bowel were also becoming inflamed, so his team decided to offer surgery. The procedure, a necrosectomy, is rarely performed these days. It involves opening the abdomen, removing as much dead tissue as possible and then irrigating the area around the pancreas for several days post-operatively. Four tubes would be left running fluid into the top of Sean's abdomen and four more lower down would drain it out again. The aim was to flush away the toxic dead pancreas as it formed and so damp down the inflammation, but operating on such fragile, inflamed tissue in a critically sick patient is fraught with hazard.

I was down in Dorset visiting my parents when Marina phoned me. The surgeon had just been round to seek Sean's consent for the procedure and both he and Marina were feeling shell-shocked. Up until that moment she had been running on autopilot. She'd been so busy with daily hospital visits and looking after Henrietta that she'd not really stopped to let it all sink in. But now the surgeon was presenting the stark facts and she and Sean had to make a terrible choice. They could continue with the present strategy, which wasn't working and on the current trajectory would leave Sean on a ventilator with multiple organ failure within a few days, or they could bite the bullet and risk surgery. The surgeon told Sean that he had at least a 30 per cent chance of dying as a result of the operation. It was an estimate, but it represented his level of concern, and as the conversation progressed Marina remembers the figure of 40 per cent creeping in. These were shocking numbers, but Sean and Marina had to know what they were agreeing to, however grim, and in the end they had to trust the people who were looking after him. Marina told me that the medical team unanimously agreed that surgery offered him the best chance, so I tried to reassure her that they were a great team of doctors and that Sean, being young and fit, was in a better position than most to withstand the stress. I knew that he would sign the form, but I can't imagine what it felt like agreeing to something that had a one-in-three chance of killing you.

The operation went well and it turned out that Sean was made of tough stuff. He spent a few days on a ventilator and then two more weeks on the ICU, but after that he was stable enough to be transferred up to a ward on the fifteenth floor of the UCH tower. I tried to visit him every time that I was in the hospital, just to break up his day (and mine), and it was during these visits that I really learnt about pancreatitis.

At medical school we learn a system for assessing a new patient. It is a medical ritual known as 'clerking' and consists of taking a history (to build a picture of the patient and what has happened to them), examination, compiling a shortlist of possible diagnoses, ordering investigations and then formulating a plan. We begin by asking what is wrong (presenting complaint) and follow this up with subsidiary questions to dig a little deeper (history of presenting complaint). We then move to other relevant information such as significant chronic health problems (past medical history), unhealthy habits (smoking, drinking, drugs), social history, family history, pets etc. The examination is also rigidly structured. We start with the hands (always approaching from the right-hand side) and then move up the arm to the eyes, mouth neck and so on. All the time we are noting clues ('clubbing' of the fingernails, jaundice in the eyes, lymph nodes in the neck etc.) as we try to elucidate the underlying diagnosis. At the end of the examination we note down all the possibilities (the differential diagnoses) and then list a stack of tests and investigations that will (hopefully) pick out one winner. It's the way doctors have done things for years – centuries, probably. Medical students go through the process meticulously, sweating as they search for the crucial diagnostic clues that they can present triumphantly to their consultant. In the modern era scans and blood tests have to some extent superseded the art of clinical inquiry, but a skilled clinician will still narrow down the possibilities and target their investigations precisely and thus economically.

In emergencies the whole rigmarole is thrown out of the window and replaced by a priority-based system of concurrent data-gathering and intervention. Helpfully, it follows the alphabet, A for airway – make sure this is open and working before moving on to B, breathing – ensure that there is adequate oxygen going in and out before C, circulation of blood, then D for disability (conscious level) etc. The order is based on what will kill you first (a blocked airway) and simplicity is the key. In a major trauma case or an acute medical emergency we can always cycle back to check A again if things become complicated or confused and immediately order is restored.

We start the history part of our clerking by asking about the patient's symptoms. People most commonly complain of pain, breathlessness, nausea, fatigue, dizziness, loss of appetite, anxiety, insomnia – all the things you'd expect – but there was one word that regularly cropped up in other people's clerkings that I never really understood – 'malaise'. I knew that it meant feeling unwell or rotten, and of course I'd felt rotten with flu and hangovers, but usually I could point to more specific symptoms such as muscle aches, headache, nausea, fever, anxiety, self-loathing or exhaustion. 'Malaise' seemed a woolly term to me, like 'nice' – until Sean educated me.

'I can only contemplate the next fifteen minutes,' he told me. 'I can't imagine feeling like this for longer. I just get through a fifteen-minute block and then I think about the fifteen after that.'

I'd experienced this with pain, but Sean wasn't in terrible pain. He just felt so awful that he had to divide his life into fifteen-minute segments and take on one at a time. I've treated the word malaise with more respect since he told me that.

Sean had another friend, a more reliable one than me, who was with him day and night: his patient-controlled analgesia (PCA) button. PCA is pain relief that patients administer to themselves. A dose of opioid (in Sean's case a powerful synthetic version called fentanyl) is delivered intravenously every time the patient presses a button. They can only get a shot every five minutes, so they can't inadvertently overdose, and the system has the dual benefits of patient autonomy and a safety feedback loop. If the drug starts to build up in their system they fall asleep and stop pressing the button, thus allowing the levels to fall again before another dose is delivered.

The fentanyl PCA was Sean's lifeline. Pancreatitis is painful, so he needed it for that, but the fentanyl did more than just relieve his pain. It removed some of his malaise and let him drift into a more pleasant existence. I think at times it gave him the strength to keep going.

We worry about patients becoming addicted to opioids. We are particularly reticent to give them a supply to take home, because it can lead to repeat prescriptions and turn into a long-term problem. This has become prescient recently as the number of people addicted to oxycodone and fentanyl soars, particularly in the United States. There is a big push to monitor and minimize opioid use, which I agree with, but whenever we discuss it I always think back to Sean. He did become dependent on fentanyl and had to wean off it slowly to avoid unpleasant withdrawal symptoms. Some people in his situation might have ended up with a long-term opioid problem, but Sean didn't. He avoids ingesting almost anything that might cause him harm, but when he needed the fentanyl, he really needed it. Should we have tried to reduce it sooner? Should we have been strict about its indication as pain relief only? Was the burden of coming off it greater than its benefit? Sean says no to all three. Most people who have opioids in hospital do not become addicts, so how careful should we be with the many to avoid problems in the few? There is, of course, a balance to be struck, but I am glad that Sean had his PCA for those weeks of malaise when he sat staring out of the window at the Post Office Tower.

Six months after his discharge from hospital, Sean was pretty much back to normal. He'd returned to work and was going for gentle runs, and Marina had started to look at property out of London. He regards himself as lucky. He survived and lives a full life (although he's never touched a drop of alcohol since). He and Marina had a second child and they did, finally, move out to the country. He says that he appreciates the simple things in life more than he used to, but he doesn't dwell on the illness. He rarely brings it up, but he and it had a profound effect on me.

Sean was the first pancreatitis patient I'd sat down with every day of their illness. For twenty minutes each day I listened to how he felt and how it was going. Not only did I get a fresh insight into what it meant to have 'malaise', I also began to understand what it means to be entirely dependent on other people. Like all patients, he trusted some nurses and doctors more than others. None was callous or dangerous, but some went the extra mile and it made all the difference. They took a little more time over things, made sure their hands were properly washed and carefully double-checked the drugs. They ensured that medications were delivered on time, that he was sleeping, that his position was optimal and that the TV remote and call bell were within easy reach. The beginning of each new shift was a nervous time for Sean as he wondered whose hands he would be in for the next twelve hours. He also told me about some of the tricky dilemmas patients face. Is it better to be pernickety about every detail and risk upsetting the staff, or easy-going and risk a mistake? You are totally reliant on the nurses, so you don't want to get a reputation – or perhaps you do. If they are worried that you might complain, might they take extra care?

We make judgements about patients and relatives every day. The lovely woman in Bed 5 who never asks for anything, the demanding son of Bed 7 who wants an update every ten minutes, the angry daughter of Bed 12 who blames us for everything, the lecherous man in Bed 27. Since Sean, I have often wondered how I would have behaved in his position. His saving grace was that he had insight. He knew when he was being finicky and the nurses knew he knew. He smiled, blamed himself and they humoured him. Perhaps there is a way to get it just right.

Sean's illness gave me a new level of empathy. Sometimes when I get into my own bed in my quiet, carpeted bedroom, with my book and wife (and occasionally child, and on particularly bad nights dog and cat), I try to imagine being instead in Bed 26 on the unit, wired up to the bleeping machinery in that dimly lit, windowless corner of Bay 3, with tubes into my stomach, airway, arteries and veins, being prodded and moved around all night. On those nights I let the dog sleep on the bed.

★

Laura was a senior trainee in intensive care and respiratory medicine and married to a colleague and close friend of mine, John. In November 2008 (shortly after Sean had finally left hospital) Laura was halfway through a year of research in Paris when she and John grabbed a last-minute deal and flew to Mauritius for a romantic break. They spent a glorious week snorkelling and sunbathing and the whole experience was only slightly marred by Laura's stomach upset on the penultimate day after some dodgy fish eaten at a game reserve. They flew back to London on a Thursday evening, tanned and refreshed, but on the Friday morning Laura developed pain in her lower back. She felt exhausted too, but she put both symptoms down to the long flight. The next day, however, she started to get pain in her hands along with pins and needles, and by the Sunday she was dragging her right foot.

Both Laura and John suspected she was suffering with Guillain–Barré syndrome (GBS), so they spoke to a friend (another doctor) who had recently recovered from it. He was reassuring: 'Yeah, sounds like GBS, but you'll be fine,' he predicted confidently. 'Milk it, though. Take some time off.'

Guillain–Barré syndrome (named after the two French neurologists, Georges Guillain and Alexandre Barré, who, along with physiologist André Strohl, fully characterized the disease in 1916) describes a set of conditions in which the body's immune system attacks the nerves or the linings of nerves and impedes their electrical impulses. The most common type in Europe, with the catchy name of acute inflammatory demyelinating polyradiculoneuropathy (AIDP), causes pins and needles, numbness, pain, loss of balance and weakness. The symptoms usually start at the extremities of the limbs and work inwards until eventually, if severe, they affect the muscles needed to swallow and breathe. The treatment is to dampen down the immune system in an attempt to halt the progress of the disease, but it is not always effective and some patients become so weak that they end up needing a ventilator.

Laura wasn't frightened, but she could tell that things were progressing quickly and she was still not sure of the diagnosis, so she decided to call her brother-in-law, a neurologist. As part of his examination he asked her to hold pieces of paper between her fingers, but she couldn't. He also tested her tendon reflexes. As most ten-year-olds know, the foot should kick out when the tendon below the knee is tapped, but Laura's did nothing. The circuit of nerves from the tendon to the spinal column and back to the leg muscles was not working. It all fitted with rapidly progressing GBS and Laura's brother-in-law suggested she go to the Royal Free Hospital's Emergency Department.

Laura remembers feeling calm as she waited to be seen that Sunday evening. She decided to write her Christmas cards, but it wasn't as easy as she'd imagined. Each one was a huge effort and her handwriting had become small and spidery. The clinical team agreed that it probably was GBS, admitted her to the medical ward and started a course of immunoglobulin (antibodies from healthy donors) to fight and dilute Laura's own antibodies, which were attacking her nerves. They also checked how deeply Laura could breathe and were reassured to discover that she could take a breath of over three litres. (Repeating this would give an objective measure of the strength of her respiratory muscles – below one litre they would start to think about putting her to sleep and taking over.)

Laura became rapidly weaker through Monday. She lost her voice and the ability to smile and by the evening she was barely able to raise her arms and legs off the bed. By Tuesday she couldn't lift her head off the pillow and the volume of her breaths was progressively falling, so they transferred her up to the ICU. That evening she started to get frightened. She was finding it harder and harder to catch her breath and by 10 p.m.

she felt as if she was drowning. She was desperate for some reassurance and a plan, but the doctors were caught up with another emergency. By midnight her breath volume was down to one litre and, by the time the team arrived, she'd started to panic. She agreed immediately with their suggestion that it was time to go onto a ventilator.

Laura woke up the next morning feeling completely calm. She had a breathing tube down her throat, which, although extremely uncomfortable for most people, didn't seem to bother her. This may have been because she had lost nerve function so couldn't cough against it, or perhaps she couldn't feel it as intensely as most people, but the important thing from her perspective was that she felt safe. She was no longer struggling for breath because the machine was doing it for her, and although she was helpless she had one-to-one attention from highly trained nurses and support from doctors and physiotherapists. A couple of days later her tube was moved from her mouth to a tracheostomy, making her ventilation both easier and more comfortable.

By now Laura could do nothing. She was a prisoner in her own body, awake but unable to move a muscle. She couldn't communicate, she couldn't breathe, she couldn't turn over or scratch her face and, on top of everything, she was in pain. The damage to the nerves of her arms and legs caused a gnawing, grinding sensation called neuropathic pain, but worse than that was the pain from her bowels. Our intestines propel food forward by contracting in synchronized ripples (peristalsis, referred to pleasingly as borborygmus when audible to the naked ear), which is under the control of the autonomic nervous system. This involuntary network of nerves also influences our heart rate, temperature control and fight-or-flight response and is often affected by GBS. In Laura's case that meant that her bowels came to a standstill. They no longer pushed forward the food and instead dilated painfully and caused her abdomen to swell like a drum. She also suffered frightening swings in her heart rate and blood pressure, and unpleasant temperature fluctuations.

For the next four weeks Laura was stuck. The nerve coatings grow back slowly (about one inch per month), and as the weakness had spread in from the tips of her limbs, so recovery would progress in the opposite direction, outwards from the centre. I visited a couple of weeks later, when she was just starting to make slow progress, and I tried to understand how she was coping. Luckily she is one of the most positive people I know, and John spent almost all of every day with her, but it wasn't easy.

She was acutely sensitive to the slightest doubt or change in mood among the clinical team, so they kept their worries away from the bedside as much as possible. They didn't lie, but they remained upbeat and that made her feel optimistic. Guillain–Barré is a disease from which people usually recover eventually, so the positive message was relatively easy to sell, but Laura reminded me how closely we are being observed by patients and relatives and the potential importance of every verbal and non-verbal cue.

She also made me reconsider how optimistic we should be with patients and their families. I had always seen it as my job to manage their (often unrealistic) expectations. I'd felt that I needed to prepare them for the worst, but in doing so perhaps I was robbing them of vital hope and the motivation to fight. It was important to be honest, but alongside that I could be upbeat and encouraging, because if I didn't think there was hope then why was I treating them at all? If I was finding it tough or depressing then perhaps I just needed to work doubly hard to ensure I didn't let that come across.

Laura described five aspects that made her ICU stay particularly tough and how she thought she'd dealt with each. The uncertainty of timescale was very hard, particularly when there was no progress from one day or even week to the next. She didn't claim to have an answer, but she felt that, overall, being a medic who had seen people recover from GBS helped – although she was also only too aware of what could go wrong. She knew that if she developed pneumonia she might die, and that was terrifying. Like Sean, she coped by limiting her horizons – surviving today was the first step, then she could think about tomorrow.

But she did not develop pneumonia or a single pressure sore, which is a testament to the quality of her care. About one in seven ventilated ICU patients develops pneumonia and a third of those die. Scrupulous attention to detail is the only way to reduce those rates. Likewise, at the time Laura was ill, one in seven ICU patients developed pressure sores. Laura was a sitting duck for both, but she got neither because her ICU nurses were meticulous about her care. Every two hours they repositioned her and checked for any marking of the skin. They ensured that she was properly fed, clean and, as far as possible, comfortable. They gave her regular mouth care and along with the physiotherapists managed the secretions in her lungs. They did everything they could to keep her safe and it worked.

Laura's next struggle was communicating. It is so often a problem for ICU patients and must drive them mad – especially when they are already feeling muddled and paranoid. A tube in the airway (be it through the mouth or the neck) and weak muscles mean that patients cannot propel air through their vocal cords so they can't speak. I have spent many hours standing at bedsides guessing the words patients are trying, ever more desperately, to mouth at me.

David was a sixty-two-year-old taxi driver recovering from pneumonia who, one morning, was clearly trying to tell me something.

'In pain?' I asked, illogically raising my voice. David had no problem with his hearing and shook his head.

'Do you feel sick?'

More head shaking.

'Thirsty?'

No.

'Need sleep?'

Another head shake, this time with a roll of the eyes.

'Too cold?'

David let his head fall back into the pillows and I reverted to platitudes.

'You're doing really well,' I reassured him. 'Would you like to try writing it down?'

Writing when you are weak, filled with sedatives and lying on your back is almost impossible. David managed a couple of legible letters but soon the shapes became spidery and trailed away. He tried again, but ended up writing words on top of other words. By now there were six or seven people around his bed, so he made one final desperate attempt to mouth a word: 'Foo . . .'

'Foo . . . d?' I guessed.

He waved me away.

Suddenly I got it.

'Football! You want to watch the football.'

He raised his eyebrows and looked at me as if to say, 'Not that hard, huh?'

My triumphant grin soon faded when I remembered that we had no TVs and the Wi-Fi on the unit was awful.

For Laura, too, communication was tough. She was awake, but also so weak that she couldn't even mouth words initially, let alone lift her hand to use a letter- or picture-board, and without John at the bedside to interpret, that period would have been unimaginable. Then, as her strength slowly improved, she began to mouth words and the nursing and medical team got better at lip-reading her until finally she could move her hands enough to use a letter-board. It took enormous patience, but it worked, and it was vital to her recovery.

Laura's next problem was passing the time. Even when the pain and other unpleasant symptoms were under control, she was left with weeks of time stretching out in front of her. She needed things to occupy her mind – a schedule. While she couldn't move at all, she interspersed the various episodes of care with reading, TV, massage and letting her imagination run wild. She craved the feeling of water against her skin and dreamt of swimming or having a bath, so the nurses washed her hair with a bucket of water. (I have images of that scene from *Out of Africa*.) The schedule worked for Laura, and just about kept her sane, but it also relied on one other crucial factor – she had to sleep through the night. In order to face each day, she needed to know that she would be unconscious that night and her team ensured that she was. They kept her as active and alert in the day as possible and then used whatever medication was required to make her sleep solidly through the night.

There is an ongoing debate about sleep in ICU. We all agree that it is vital for sanity and recovery, but whether we should aim to use non-pharmacological methods as far as possible and accept fewer hours of potentially higher quality 'natural' sleep, or be more liberal with the hypnotic drugs and prioritize longer periods of unconsciousness, remains contentious. I hate the word 'natural' when it is used to imply health or, worse, moral superiority, but even I had bought into the natural-sleep argument (despite a lack of convincing scientific evidence) – until Laura's experience made me reconsider. Her doctors didn't give her more medication than was necessary, but they gave her enough to ensure that she slept through the night. The pharmacologically assisted sleep seemed restorative to her, it ate up hours and, most importantly, the knowledge that she'd be unconscious from 10 p.m. to 7 a.m. gave her the strength to carry on.

The lowest point for Laura was when she stepped down from ICU to the general ward. We might think of this as a moment of triumph, a big step towards recovery, but when patients come to ICU for a second time they are often terrified of leaving because they know that when they do the nurse-to-patient ratio will drop dramatically, often from 1:1 to 1:8. By the time Laura was transferred from ICU her tracheostomy had been removed and she could breathe for herself, but she was still being fed through a tube and she was still too weak to turn over in bed or raise her hand to her face. She felt abandoned and frightened. She was waiting for a specialist neuro-rehabilitation bed at the National Hospital for Neurology and Neurosciences in Queens Square and was terrified that she'd suffer a complication, become too unwell to go and lose her slot. She felt more vulnerable than ever.

But again the nurses kept her free from complications, she made it to rehab and twelve weeks later, at the end of April 2009, she went home. It was almost six months since she'd noticed her first symptom, but still her recovery was far from complete. She needed a carer to help her get up, dressed and down the stairs in the morning, crockery regularly slipped between her fingers and smashed on the floor, and when she took short walks outside with a stick she often stumbled or fell and was both embarrassed and angry when people presumed that she was drunk. But she was delighted to be home.

In October 2009, eleven months after her fateful trip to Maur-itius, Laura returned to work. Twelve years later she still has foot drop* and a slightly weak left hand, but she cycles and

---

* Foot drop describes the inability to bend up the forefoot at the ankle; think John Thaw in *Inspector Morse*.

swims, has had three children and is a consultant respiratory physician and academic at the Royal Brompton Hospital as well as a successful artist.

She says that now there is enough distance from her illness to talk about it dispassionately, but for five years the subject conjured all sorts of powerful emotions. Her husband was also profoundly affected. It is easy to forget what the relatives go through, but watching your spouse so helpless and vulnerable for so long has a deep and lasting impact. Often relatives are strong through the acute illness but then collapse when their loved ones start to get better, and when I interviewed them for this book, John found the episode much harder to talk about than Laura did.

On one level I already knew everything that Sean and Laura told me about being an ICU patient. I've met thousands of them. I've asked them how they are feeling, sympathized with them and tried to imagine myself in their position. I've read about the psychological impact of a stay on ICU; the high levels of ongoing anxiety and depression, the number of patients who never make it back to work and the impact on the people around them. And yet Sean and Laura made me understand these things in a different, more profound way, because I knew them and their families before they were ill. I could talk to them as friends (not just as a doctor) without worrying about causing offence. I saw how the experience changed them and I watched them reclaim their lives.

They emphasized the importance of things like sleep and malaise to ICU patients and the impact of the clinicians' demeanour, but they also broke down barriers that I hadn't realized were there and brought me closer to the other patients. Up until then there'd been a reassuring distance between us. Most of the patients were either significantly older than I was or terribly unlucky. I felt sorry for them, but also guiltily smug about my own health and youth. Now two previously fit friends, both younger than me, had been struck down with critical illness and one had nearly died. I didn't feel smug any more, I felt middle-aged and vulnerable and my attitude shifted. I found it harder to judge when cases had become futile and I took longer to come to conclusions and to make decisions. I questioned 'prognostic truths' I'd taken for granted, and when I did make decisions they weighed on me more heavily.

I also decided it was time to adopt a more healthy lifestyle.

7. Beds

I was already restless when the alarm went off at 6.30 on the morning of 16 December 2014. The last call I'd received had been at 3 a.m., but it had left me unsettled. Mark, a patient I'd recently discharged to the general ward, was on his way back to the unit. He was a man in his forties who'd received a bone-marrow transplant to treat his leukaemia just over three weeks previously and was still profoundly immunosuppressed. He'd been in ICU the first time with neutropenic sepsis,* so we'd given him drugs to support his blood pressure, antibiotics and high-flow oxygen, but he had got away without needing a ventilator. I'd discharged him on 14 December, but last night he'd felt faint and vomited. Some of the vomit had gone into his lungs and his oxygen levels had plummeted, so the anaesthetists had put him to sleep, intubated him and brought him back to the ICU via the CT scanner. Now he was sicker than ever.

Perhaps I had discharged him too soon.

'I swear I'll go mad if I have to spend another night in here,' Mark had pleaded two days ago. He'd been in Side Room 5, a run-of-the-mill ICU single room – eight feet by ten, garish strip lighting, lots of equipment, pink and green circles on the walls, no Wi-Fi and a window behind his head that looked out onto the Euston Road. My plan had been to keep him for

---

* It takes a few weeks for the transplanted bone marrow to start producing white blood cells. Before then the patients lack the cells required to fight off bacteria, neutrophils. Unsurprisingly during this period they are at high risk of blood infections – 'neutropenic sepsis'.

another day, but his cell count was beginning to improve and I'd felt desperately sorry for him. He had two daughters aged four and six that he'd not seen since the transplant. His wife didn't want to bring them to ICU.

The registrar had texted back at 4 a.m. to say that Mark was now safely settled into Side Room 4 on the ICU – identical to Side Room 5 except a few feet closer to Tottenham Court Road.

'Thanks,' I'd replied and then drifted off to sleep.

Now all thirty-five ICU beds were full.

As I shuffled into the bathroom a few hours later I thought about the day ahead. Quick catch-up with the night team at 7.45, team brief with the nurses at 8 a.m., formal handover from the night doctors 8.05 to 9 o'clock, then catch up with the nurse in charge about beds (I was still the on-call ICU consultant and 'gate keeper' for the next twenty-four hours) and then a very brief preliminary ward round before the big bed meeting at 9.30. Tish walked sleepily into the bathroom behind me.

'Sorry about all the calls,' I mumbled through my toothbrush.

'What calls?' she yawned. I don't know how she does it. My phone must have rung six times since midnight. 'Are you going to be able to come tonight?'

Tish was reading at a charity carol concert that evening. I'd sent a group message to my consultant colleagues to see if anyone could cover, but it was the same night as the ICU Christmas party.

'What time?'

'Seven thirty.'

'I'll try,' I said.

'I could take your brother?'

'Oh, OK.'

I felt an unjustified pang of irritation. It would be a beautiful carol concert and that was my ticket, not his. I wasn't working, I was on call. I was supposed to leave the hospital at 6.30 and then be available for advice (and to return if necessary), so I should, by the letter of the law, be able to go to the concert.

'When are you reading?'

'Dunno.'

'Take my brother. I'm sorry.'

When I am on call and trying to be somewhere at a particular time, I become agitated and glance at the clock every ten minutes for about two hours before the deadline. If I just focused on the patients for those two hours I'd not only do a better job, I'd also be more likely to make it to the event, but I can't help trying to manipulate the day to fit my plans. Usually I fail, but if I do get to the film or play or match, I then spend a good proportion of it worrying about whether I've got enough phone reception and how easily I can slip away when the inevitable call comes. Text messaging is a partial solution, but it results in a lot of tutting at the National Theatre, so I end up texting bent down below the seat pretending to look for my glasses. It does not make for a relaxing night out.

Tish should definitely take my brother.

She put a hand on my shoulder before shivering and heading back to the bedroom.

It took a minute for anyone to look up. Two registrars, an SHO and the ICU nurse in charge overnight were all sitting behind reception. The SHO, wearing a hoodie over her scrubs, was typing up notes, the nurse in charge was trying to work out how to allocate the incoming day shift, one registrar was idly scratching his stubble and grazing from a bag of Haribo and the other was stretched rigidly across his chair, like one end of a seesaw, with his head nestled neatly into a pigeon hole, asleep. I leant in over the front desk.

'Dr Down. Good morning.' The SHO was the first to spot me.

'Hi, busy night?' It was somewhere between a question and a statement, an attempt to acknowledge the hard work they'd put in without undermining their ownership of the experience.

'Yeah.' The registrar who'd nodded off, Sam, was now sitting forward, rubbing his eyes and looking unnecessarily embarrassed. I asked about Mark. 'Sorry. Umm, yeah . . . all OK-ish. He's not too bad. They're just getting the lines in.'

'Can you get the scan report up?'

'Sure; nothing dramatic.'

I turned to Stephen, the nurse in charge.

'And that's our last bed, yeah?'

'We have one more physical bed, but the day-shift staffing is not good.'

'Mr Heath – Bed 8 – died.' The SHO clarified.

Mr Heath was an eighty-three-year-old with a pneumonia on the background of smoking-induced chronic lung disease who the day before had moved to a palliative pathway.

'Family in?'

'Wife and son, both very grateful.'

'How many electives to come in from theatres?'

'Ten,' Stephen said, glancing down at his sheet of paper.

'And there are two more sickies on the ward,' Sam added.*
'Oh, and there's one who might need to come from ED.'

'And discharges?'

---

* 'Sicky' is the term we use for patients who are causing concern – 'dodgy looking' being an equally highbrow alternative. The vernacular of clinicians is an odd combination of technical terminology, acronyms and cheerfully brutal similes and metaphors – 'The sickie with the ACS is looking much more chipper'; 'Lorna, the strongyloides in Bed 4, has fallen in a heap'; 'With the furosemide she's started peeing like a racehorse' etc. It's just the way medics have always spoken.

'Eight, possibly nine ready, but I've only been given four beds. The wards are heaving.'

'Right.'

'I've said yes to three.' Stephen was studying another piece of paper now. 'We'll have to discuss the rest at the nine-thirty meeting.'

'Can't wait.'

It was a typical December Tuesday. As ever, we were trying to deal with the standard winter pressures (flu, pneumonia, broken hips etc.), while also accommodating a full programme of major elective surgery. First, we had to decide who could leave the safety and security of the ICU to fend for themselves in the less well-staffed general wards, and then we needed to find them the right type of bed. Some needed a specialist bed, some a side room and some an extra nurse. Next, we had to decide how many ICU beds to keep for the 'sickies' on the wards and the 'potentials' through the ED and then, finally, to select which of the ten elective surgical candidates should get the remaining ICU beds.

Stephen had already said yes to three cancer patients: a woman having a fourteen-hour throat operation, a man in for a six-hour oesophagus resection and a woman having her womb and a section of bowel removed. That left two major redo hip replacements on patients with complex medical problems, two major bowel resections (cancer again), one frail woman with a broken hip, one man to have lasering of a recurrent lesion in his windpipe, a young woman scheduled to have a gastric bypass for obesity – plus Dan's two 'sickies' on the ward and a 'possibility' in the Emergency Department.

I had two unallocated ICU beds left to play with (with a possible further four or five more to come later) and between seven and ten people trying to get into them. I also needed to keep at least one (ideally two) beds free for unexpected emergencies, so in the end I had between two and seven beds for between nine and twelve patients. My head was hurting already. Many things might change through the day, but two things were clear: I didn't have enough beds for everyone and I had to give the impression that I had a plan. It's been the same for the last fifteen years. Sometimes I feel in control and sometimes I feel like the plaything of some sadistic supernatural bed-saboteur.

After the handover I did a whistle-stop ward round to see if there was any opportunity to discharge people and clear beds. One patient who'd had a gullet resection two days before looked very well. He was sitting out of bed, comfortable and chatting away, but it's a high-risk operation and the most likely time for a complication would be on day three or four. On ICU any deterioration would be picked up quickly, but on the ward it might not be noticed for several crucial hours. Another man in his seventies was recovering from pneumonia. He'd come off the ventilator the previous evening and was holding his own, but his breathing was shallow and he had spiked a fever an hour ago. He just didn't look right. If he went to the ward he might be fine, but equally he might fall in a heap and be back with us within twenty-four hours – and I didn't need another readmission.

I was loath to discharge either of these, so what about at the other end of the spectrum? Was anyone likely to die today? Was there anyone whose treatment had become futile? No one was at death's door, but there was a patient whose prognosis looked bleak. He was a sixty-two-year-old who had suffered a cardiac arrest at home after a blood clot had lodged in his lungs five days previously. He'd had a prolonged period of CPR and suffered significant brain injury from lack of oxygen. He showed little sign of waking up, despite receiving no sedation for the last three days, but he was occasionally coughing against the ventilator, so he was not brain dead.* Although none of us felt optimistic, it was too early to know exactly how much his brain might improve in the longer term and his family were still desperately hoping he'd wake up.

'First, do no harm' is one of the guiding principles of medicine, and moving any of these patients risked doing just that. If they had been lower risk, I might have considered gambling and discharging one of the two patients who was almost ready for the ward in order to make way for elective surgery, but I would never withdraw treatment on a patient who had a poor but not yet hopeless prognosis for that reason. No intensivist I know would. We might have different thresholds for deciding when a case is hopeless, but none of us would allow that judgement to be influenced by the pressure for beds.

The distinction between these two groups makes sense to me emotionally, because the patient who is discharged early and then deteriorates can always come back to ICU. Usually they will be 'rescued' and recover, but even if they die it will be put down to a multitude of factors – not just the fact that I sent them out a bit early. But a very sick patient that I discharge who as a result gets palliated will definitely die. There is a clear cause and effect. I might argue that they would have died anyway, but I can't get away from the fact that by discharging them I made that a certainty.

The first of these two options seems far more attractive, but I am not sure that my logic stands up to scrutiny. In effect, I am saying that I am happy to reduce someone's chance of surviving from say 95 per cent to 85 per cent, but not from 10 per cent to 0 per cent – and that is before we even consider issues such as the length and quality of their future life. The recovering patient

* Brain death describes a state in which the primitive part of the brain, the brain stem, has permanently stopped functioning (see Chapter 9).

might miss out on twenty years of a full active life, whereas the 'probably palliative' one may at best lose a few months.

A third option would be to move one of our most stable patients to a less busy ICU in another hospital. The difficulty with this is that the individual who moves faces the potential harm of the transfer, but no benefit. Even in a crisis many intensivists are happier to transfer a patient who needs ICU, but has not yet secured a bed, than one already in an ICU bed. The former has something to gain from the transfer, i.e. an ICU bed, whereas the latter risks harm for no benefit. But I believe that both have equal right to future ICU care (whatever their current circumstance) so the choice should be made purely on the relative risks of the two transfers. Many relatives and colleagues disagree, however, and I suspect that if it was my wife who was to be evicted from an ICU and carted ten miles across London in the back of a draughty ambulance, I might well disagree with myself.

In the event, all our local ICUs were in a similar position to us that day, so transfer was not a viable option; we still had two to seven beds for nine to twelve patients and were left with three broad alternatives. We could cancel operations, we could downgrade patients from ICU care to ward care post-operatively or we could overbook the unit and hope for the best. Depending on how the day panned out, we'd then deal with the problem later by converting some recovery beds into a pop-up ICU for the night or, if absolutely necessary, transferring people (a long way) out of the hospital.

By the time I sat down for the 9.30 bed meeting I was irritable. At this stage of the day I am always twitchy because I want to get on with reviewing my patients, and that morning I was particularly distracted by Mark, our overnight readmission. I'd only glanced at him briefly, but he didn't look good and I couldn't shake off the feeling that I was responsible. There was nothing I could do about it now, though, so I tried to push him to the back of my mind. I tried, but I knew that I'd actually stop worrying about him only when and if he started to improve again. More time and energy spent on the impossible daily bed puzzle was the last thing I needed, but as it happened I received a pleasant surprise. The bed managers had discovered a few more ward beds and only one of the three possible emergencies needed to come to ICU.

Now we had ten patients trying to get into seven beds. We were getting closer. Should we downgrade? Should we cancel? Should we wing it and kick the problem down the road?

The obvious patient to cancel was the bariatric case. She had a benign disease, she'd been morbidly obese for years and there was always the other option – lifestyle change. On the other hand she had been cancelled twice already and she was desperate for surgery. Every day she suffered the complications of her obesity: diabetes, high blood pressure, sleep apnoea and depression. All these conditions would lead to further complications and some of those would be life threatening. And could she really lose the weight herself? It is so easy to be judgemental and assume so, but the evidence would suggest otherwise. The physiology and psychology of tackling morbid obesity are far more complex than 'eating less and moving around more'. But she didn't have cancer and she wasn't in constant pain from a failing hip prosthesis so it might be argued that her surgery was less time critical. Then again, the bed situation would probably be no different next week or the week after. Should her procedure continue to be postponed indefinitely to make way for more seriously ill patients? She could end up waiting months, by which time her own life might be in danger.

Perhaps the solution was to go ahead with her surgery, but send her to the normal ward post-op. She was booked for ICU because she had sleep apnoea and used a CPAP machine every night.* Sleep apnoea is a condition in which the throat closes when the patient falls asleep due to the drop in muscle tone. Snorers partially occlude their throats, making their breathing noisy, but if the airway blocks completely the person stops breathing. It is only when the oxygen tension in the blood dips to a level low enough to stimulate arousal that they stir, the muscle tone increases and they take a huge breath. The pauses between breaths can be alarming for partners (who commonly shout '*Breathe!*' at their loved one, or kick them), but intervention is not only to improve marital harmony: if left untreated, sleep apnoea can have serious medical consequences. Patients never get a good night's sleep because they are constantly having to 'almost' wake up to breathe. Consequently they are left somnolent in the day, the most severe cases living their whole lives in a stuporous twilight zone. The low oxygen tension also makes the blood vessels in the lungs constrict. That puts pressure on the right side of the heart (the side that pumps the blood to the lungs), which then fails, resulting in back pressure and accumulation of fluid in the tissues (swollen legs). Eventually, the big failing right heart puts pressure on the left heart and the whole heart–lung unit breaks down. All from some snoring that got out of hand.

The mainstays of treatment are weight loss and nocturnal CPAP, but the CPAP devices are uncomfortable and noisy and many patients do not tolerate them. Those who do, however, report the life-changing benefits of the first good night's sleep they have had for years.

---

* A CPAP, or continuous positive airway pressure machine, delivers constant positive pressure to the patient's face and thus airways via a mask or hood and blows them open – like sticking your head out of the car window on the motorway.

Our hospital policy is to admit all patients who use CPAP to ICU after major surgery, because they are not only at risk of blocking their airways after an anaesthetic but are also acutely sensitive to opioids and can stop breathing after relatively small doses. I was not going to mess with hospital policy, so she would either get an ICU bed or be cancelled.

The two remaining cancer patients (the bowel resections) were the clinical priorities, so the only question for them was did they *have* to go to ICU or could they go straight back to the ward?

The logic for admitting them was to keep a close eye on their physiology straight after the operation, avoid problems and treat those that did occur promptly. Studies have shown that early post-operative complications affect patients' chances of dying for years afterwards, so there is a strong argument for trying to avoid them, but where do you draw the line? A huge number of people might have a marginal gain from a night on ICU after their operation, but the magnitude of that gain depends both on the size of the operation and the fitness of the patient. I am fifty-one years old. If I had the right side of my colon removed (a relatively safe bowel operation) my chances of an uncomplicated recovery would be increased by a night in ICU and, in the private sector, I would get one automatically. However, I have no chronic health conditions and I go for a run or a swim most days so my baseline risk of complications is low. I would be fine going straight back to a normal ward, perhaps 95 per cent of the time. A night on ICU might increase that to, say, 98 per cent. When I am sixty-one and speed-walking rather than running, those percentages might fall to 90 per cent and 95 per cent and if I make it to seventy-one and am shuffling along with a pot belly and sore hips they might fall to 75 per cent and 85 per cent. At what point should I stop taking my chances and be offered a precious ICU bed?

We have scoring systems to evaluate the risks for different groups of patients undergoing different operations, and on that day one bowel resection had an estimated mortality of 11 per cent whereas the other's was only 5 per cent, so I gave my first ICU bed to the former. I didn't look more closely at their relative urgency because we had to get on with it, but I did reconsider the patients we'd already given the green light to – particularly the woman with throat cancer. The decision about her had been deemed easy because she would be ventilated for twenty-four hours so couldn't be looked after on the normal ward, and she was also having cancer surgery so she was a slam dunk – the top priority. Or was she? Her chances of surviving the cancer for another year, even with successful surgery, were only 30 per cent. Fifty years of smoking and drinking meant that the risk of post-operative complications was high and a prolonged stay on ICU likely. Proceeding with her surgery might mean delaying several other cases over the next few days who could have sequentially occupied her bed. She might well die in the next year for unrelated reasons. Did she really trump the other cancers, or even the bariatric patient? In terms of potential QUALYs (quality-adjusted life years) gained, the bariatric patient would win hands down. It was too late to worry about that now, though, the throat operation was already well under way. (*Focus, Jim. Come on!*)

I was now left with the second bowel cancer, the two redo hips, the emergency fractured hip, the bariatric case, the windpipe lasering and the need to keep one emergency bed (ideally, two). I had five beds to play with, but took that down to three to keep my emergency beds. Six cases for three beds. Now we were at the sharp end.

The mortality risks of the two revision hips was calculated to be 6 per cent and 9 per cent (the second being older with a very poor heart), the colon cancer 5 per cent and the fractured hip

7 per cent. The patient for lasering might not be able to breathe after the procedure so, if done, he had to come to ICU.

I didn't know the right answer. Perhaps there wasn't one. In a few hours the situation could be very different (for better or worse) and my decision (whatever it was) seem inspired or foolish. I decided to cancel the bariatric case, proceed with the colon-cancer patient, the fractured hip and one of the two redo hips and put the other hip and the laser case on hold. I felt relatively confident that the first hip and either the fracture or the colon-cancer resection would sail through, look peachy at the end of surgery and be able to go back to the normal ward, at which point we *should* be able to go ahead with some others . . . as long as the Emergency Department didn't go mad; or the wards.

I felt bad about the bariatric patient, but just as I was reconsidering my decision the whole thing was taken out of my hands. A message came through that one of the surgical wards had an outbreak of the vomiting and diarrhoea bug norovirus and would be closing fifteen beds. All elective non-cancer cases requiring an inpatient bed that had not already started would have to be postponed.

After all that.

On the plus side, we'd do all the cancer cases and the decisions were now made, so we could tell the patients straight away and I could get on with my job. The theatre staff could also get on with some emergencies rather than sit around all day waiting for a decision and we could ditch the usual follow-up meeting at lunchtime. Many at the 9.30 meeting would have to meet again at 3 p.m. to talk about the next day, but not me, thank God.

As I write this down it seems extraordinary that such important decisions about people's lives are made in such a last-minute and ad hoc fashion, but they are – and not occasionally but every day, as tens of thousands of patients who have had their operations postponed will confirm. And compared to many hospitals, at UCH we have good ICU capacity.

Bed juggling is not a glamorous or exciting part of the job, but it takes up a huge amount of our time and will continue to do so for as long as we work in an unpredictable and over-stretched system. While emergencies compete with elective cases and we run at over 90 per cent capacity, the daily tussles will go on. Perhaps that is as it should be. Patients may get cancelled on the day, but no one can claim that we are not sweating the system. They might, however, question whether we are working as safely, compassionately and efficiently as possible, and whether we are using the ICU beds in the fairest and most efficacious way. Like all hospitals, we have spent the last ten years searching for solutions. We have hired frighteningly young management consultants to brainstorm and 'unlock fresh ideas'. We have assembled teams who have shifted patients from their beds into hurriedly built discharge lounges. We have purchased electronic 'live-bed-state technology' to show everyone what is (or isn't) happening minute by minute across the hospital and we have appointed Tsars of flow because 'If we could just sort out the flow our troubles would be over.'

And with each innovation there has been a palpable sense of hope, but by the following autumn the familiar problems have recurred. And the next autumn and the one after that. The Covid pandemic shone a light on ICU bed capacity, but this is nothing new. The UK has had one of the lowest rates of ICU beds per head of population in Europe for years and now, after Brexit, staffing the beds we do have has become increasingly challenging. Our ICU used to be a smorgasbord of young vibrant European nursing and medical talent. They relished the opportunity to spend a few years discovering London (and the NHS) during their twenties. While some stayed on, most returned home to settle in more affordable locations, but during their time here they not only filled vital vacancies, they also enriched our working environment. It has been heartbreaking to see their numbers fall away.

This might all be manageable if the demand through the year was constant, but, of course, it isn't. Winter is always busier, every year without fail, because of flu and other seasonal infections. People have talked about giving ICU staff annualized contracts so more of them are around at the busier times, which seems an appealing idea, because many staff might enjoy long summer holidays, but we would also need more physical ICU beds in the winter. Flexing down elective surgery in winter is equally problematic because the pressure to meet surgical waiting-time targets is relentless and idle operating theatres, scrub staff, anaesthetists and surgeons are expensive.

We could divide hospitals into hot (emergency) and cold (elective) sites. That way the two groups of patients would never compete for the same beds and in the cold sites planning could be more precise. Where I work there are three hospitals within a three-mile radius, all with emergency departments, ICUs and elective operating. We could make one of them pure emergency and the other two elective. Instead of three emergency departments there would be one, and staff could do blocks (say a week) of emergency work and then move back to the elective hospitals for three weeks. This is unlikely to happen because people don't like change, both the staff and the patients feel strong allegiance to their own hospital, the merger and transformation would be fiendishly complex and there is too much local political pressure to keep all three emergency departments open.

I thought with my elective/emergency split I'd nailed it and I swanned around smugly complaining that no one was politically brave enough to do the right thing. But the Covid pandemic changed my perspective because it made me appreciate how vital it is for people to visit their loved ones in hospital.

Previously this had been way down my priority list and, shamefully, I'd rather taken it for granted, but having lived through a time when families couldn't come in, the importance of visiting has really hit home. Patients and their families need to see each other. Such a division might be feasible for hospitals in close proximity, but if relatives have to undertake a lengthy expensive round trip to visit then, of course, they won't come as often. My mother was in a nursing home three hours' drive from where I live. I visited 'when I could'. Of course, I could have visited more often, but I had a job and kids and commitments and excuses. If she'd been twenty minutes away I would have visited a lot more. The convenience of local hospitals is not like the convenience of a TV remote control, it has a real impact on what is often the most frightening and difficult period of people's lives.

Covid has at least improved collaboration among hospitals. We have always helped each other out with beds, but the system had been haphazard. Before the pandemic we rang around other units when we needed a bed and begged. All the power lay with the receiving ICU consultant and the rules of engagement were open to interpretation. We'd usually try to help each other, but the natural instinct was to protect your own patch. No one wanted to risk pushing their own unit into a bed crisis and there was always the anxiety that you might be accepting the heart-sink patient with the hopeless prognosis and the litigious family. One of those can be around for weeks and bring down the morale of the whole ICU.

But the pandemic changed all that. Now there are phone calls and endless WhatsApp messages across our sector every day to make sure that centres with capacity are using our new bespoke transfer service to offload those under the most pressure. The goal is to use the region's ICU bed base equitably and so far it is working. It's no help when we're all overwhelmed, but it does seem to be largely doing what splitting elective and emergency work between hospitals would have done.

Telling patients that their operations will not be going ahead is an unpleasant task, but it is only my responsibility when we are postponing for clinical reasons. I have the luxury of being able to use phrases such as 'it is for your safety' and 'I couldn't live with myself if something went wrong', which usually placate patients, but when the cancellation is for non-clinical reasons the reaction is less predictable. Usually the surgeons tell their own patients because they have an established relationship, but sometimes the grim task falls to mid-level NHS managers. These are the people I feel sorry for. Many colleagues argue that the cause of the postponement is 'managerial', so the managers should witness the result of their inadequacies and deal with the ensuing anger and despair, but the truth is that the managers have an impossible task. They have to balance the books, make sure that as many patients as possible get treated, deal with difficult clinicians and comply with national standards and policies, while taking the blame for almost everything. How many times have we heard that 'there are far too many NHS managers at the expense of front-line staff', as if somehow they are a superfluous or even malevolent workforce holding back the doctors and nurses. Of course, some of them are better than others, but as a group I've found them to be talented, capable, professional and just as devoted to the NHS as the clinicians.

That day, the surgeon told the bariatric patient that she had yet again been postponed and her reaction was almost apologetic – as if it was shameful that she needed the operation in the first place when the NHS was clearly under so much pressure. The manager for surgery, however, had a very different experience with one of the patients due for a redo hip operation. He was outraged and livid. He'd paid taxes all his life, had rearranged several overseas business trips and was due to go on holiday to the Maldives in two months. Would the NHS be refunding him for his holiday costs? He took the manager's details and promised he'd be taking this further. UCH, and this 'administrator' in particular, had not heard the end of it. If he treated his clients in this abominable way he'd be bankrupt within a week.

The manager apologized again and showed great restraint in not pointing out that, bankrupt or not, the next available opportunity for him to have his surgery would probably be long after his trip to the Maldives.

My mood perked up considerably on the evening ward round when we got to Bed 4. Mark had improved significantly and at this rate he would be off the ventilator within forty-eight hours. I felt a weight lift from my shoulders as I gave his wife the good news, but on the bus home that evening I wondered whether we could do all of this better. My colleague Steve has spent the last few years developing models to forecast the flow of patients around the hospital. When these come to fruition they will help us to make predictions, but they'll never tell us how many people are going to become critically sick in the community on any given week. We will still be making difficult decisions about bed allocation on a daily basis.

That night two ICU patients died, one woke up from a drug overdose and self-discharged and there were, unbelievably, no admissions from the Emergency Department. I could have taken all the surgical patients after all, but by then they were back home, busy trying to rearrange their lives and expectations and in one case writing a strongly worded letter to our chief executive.

8.   Blame

'Hi, Jim, sorry to bother you.'

'No problem.' I pushed myself up the pillows and rubbed my eyes.

'Do you know Fergus in Bed 24?'

'Yes, pneumonia and ACS, the one Dan extubated this afternoon.'

'Yeah. He's not looking so good.'

'OK.'

'Oxygen sats in the high eighties on 80 per cent oxygen, opti-flow, he's tachypnoeic and his chest sounds . . . grim.'

It was just before midnight on 12 November 2015. I was four days into my week of ICU, my third night on call. I'd been deeply asleep because the previous night had been busy. Noth-ing too complicated, but there'd been regular admissions between midnight and 6 a.m.: a diabetic coma, a mixed drug overdose and a bad asthma attack. I'd spent a lot of that night on the phone, but tonight's discussion with the ICU registrar, Luke, at 10.30 p.m. had been encouraging. The patients on the unit were behaving themselves, the wards were quiet and there was nothing terrible in the ED. I'd forgotten to ask specifically about Fergus, but Luke hadn't mentioned him and I'd stupidly allowed myself to visualize the finish line. A good sleep tonight, one more day on the unit tomorrow and I'd be free. Back then only one consultant covered the ICU at the weekend, which was pretty hideous, but this wasn't my weekend. I was off to a university reunion, where I'd immediately slip back into my designated role of energetic, sarcastic, beer-soaked twenty-one-year-old. We were due to meet in an Elizabethan Landmark Trust property in North Somerset and planned to spend the weekend wandering through the soggy countryside and complaining about middle age. We would cook stodgy food, relive medical-school indiscretions and then drift into a booze-assisted slumber. I couldn't wait.

Fergus was sixty-one years old but physiologically much older. He'd smoked twenty a day since his late teens and been admitted to the unit three times over the last two years with pneumonia. Twice we'd had to sedate and ventilate him, each time with a sense of foreboding, but both times he'd confounded us, bounced back and gone home. This time, however, as well as his usual pneumonia he'd suffered an acute coronary syndrome,* which had left his heart weakened. He'd been on the ventilator for two weeks, but over the last four days he had improved, responding to antibiotics and heart-failure medication, and my colleague Dan had spotted a window. The previous morning when they'd turned down the sedation, he'd obeyed commands and his oxygen requirements were only 40 per cent. This might be the one chance to take him off the ventilator and get the breathing tube out. It was risky, because he still had a lot of secretions in his lungs, but by tomorrow he could well be worse again: a bit weaker, a bit more confused and brewing a new infection. The alternative was to exchange the tube through the mouth for a tracheostomy (more comfortable and easier to breathe through) and then wean him slowly from the ventilator over the next week or two, but Dan had decided to take the chance and pull the tube. Putting in a trachey was not without risks, so if we could get away without it – great. If Dan's plan

* Acute coronary syndrome (ACS) is a blockage to one of the blood vessels to the heart muscle – a heart attack.

didn't work he'd just put Fergus back to sleep, put a tube back down and tee up a trachey for the next day.

On the afternoon ward round, Fergus had looked OK . . . ish. He was awake and in good spirits, giving us a strong thumbs-up when we asked how he felt, but his cough lacked bite (reminding me of one of those fududud vacuum cleaners from the 1970s) and he was reliant on high-flow oxygen. He wasn't breathing particularly fast, which was encouraging, but every breath looked hard work.

'I think he'll do,' Dan predicted, spotting me loitering a little longer at the bedside. 'He's only been off the vent for an hour.'

'Hmm.' I glanced at the laminated airway plan behind Fergus's bed. 'Easy intubation?'

'Yeah.' Dan hesitated. 'Well, he was awkward, I think, but fine. The notes are a bit sketchy, grade 2b.'

Every patient on the unit has an 'airway plan' stuck to the wall behind their bed that tells us which technique to use should we need to put a breathing tube down in a hurry. Usually this involves following the standard algorithm, and in the vast majority of cases it all goes smoothly. We put the patient to sleep, paralyse them and then look down into the throat with our laryngoscope, get a beautiful view of the whole of the vocal cords (a grade 1 view) and slip our breathing tube between them and into the trachea. Occasionally, however, the anatomy conspires against us and, rather than a view of the whole of the vocal cords, we see just part of them (grade 2 to 2b if we can see only the very back) or just the flap of tissue above them (the epiglottis, grade 3) or none of the above (grade 4). When we can't see where to put the tube, life is more difficult, but that is fine as long as we can take out the laryngoscope and ventilate the lungs via a tight-fitting mask over the nose and mouth, which we usually can. But, very occasionally, we can't do that either. At this point the patient's oxygen levels usually start to drop and we begin to feel a bit twitchy, but even then, we've still got options. We can try a different device that sits at the back of the throat (a laryngeal mask) and ventilate through that, we can ask a more senior person to have a go at intubating, we can try a different laryngoscope, we can sometimes wake the patient up and, if all else fails, we can make a hole in the neck and attempt to insert a breathing tube into the trachea that way. As you might imagine, that's very much the last resort.

We get hints from looking at a patient as to whether any or all of these procedures might be difficult. We ask them to open their mouths wide and to bend their heads forward and back and we feel the front of the throat. We prefer clean-shaven patients with huge mouths, small solid teeth or no teeth at all, long, slim, bendy necks and a strong jawline.

All these features build a picture, but it's not definitive. We don't actually know if we will be able to insert a breathing tube or ventilate a patient until we put them to sleep, paralyse them and try. It is reassuring if they have been anaesthetized previously without incident, but things can change over time.

Fergus had buck teeth, a short thick neck and a beard.

'Can you put your chin on your chest and then look up at the ceiling?' I asked.

He looked down and then up, but his head didn't move very much.

'Can you open your mouth for me?'

Fergus dutifully opened his mouth, but not wide. It was a far cry from Bart screaming on *The Simpsons*. There was no sign of the wobbly bit at the back of his mouth (the uvula).

'He's getting better,' Dan reassured me. 'The physios are coming back to clear some more secretions. He'll be fine.'

And we moved on.

Six hours later, Fergus was clearly not fine.

'Did the physios come?' I asked, speaking quietly so as not to disturb Tish.

'I don't know, sorry,' Luke replied. 'Not since I've been here.'

'What does his chest sound like?'

'Full of secretions. He's coughing, but he just can't clear them, and he looks knackered.'

'OK,' I sighed, 'I guess we'll have to re-tube him.'

'I'm getting the stuff together now.'

'He was OK last time, I gather, but have you got another pair of hands?'

'Yeah, I've called the anaesthetic reg who's post-CCT. And Tom's the other ICU reg, I think he's peri-CCT as well.'*

These were fully qualified doctors ready to apply for consultant posts.

'Sounds good; call me if you're not happy.'

'Thanks. Sure.'

I put the phone back on my bedside table and sat staring at the small crack of light between the bedroom curtains. Perhaps I should just go in. I hadn't liked the look of Fergus's airway and I was the consultant, so I was ultimately responsible (even if I was miles away in my bedroom) – but Fergus had been intubated without too much difficulty last time and there were two fully qualified anaesthetists on site. I couldn't go in for every intubation, and they'd be just as good as me, probably better. It would take me twenty-five minutes to get there, by which time they would have sorted it all out. They were senior, skilled and experienced people – but . . . Was the registrar really happy? He'd said so, but I'd sensed something in the tone of his voice. Not panic, or anger – it was difficult to pinpoint, but I felt

---

* CCT stands for Certificate of Completion of Training. 'Peri-CCT' is used of someone who is about to complete their training.

uneasy. Then again, I often feel uneasy. Perhaps I was just being paranoid.

I sat fidgeting for fifteen minutes, my mind flitting around random topics:

If I'm up all night, should I drive to Somerset tomorrow evening?
I should give up meat; New Year's resolution.
I wonder if there's a train?
'No more bacon though? . . . I'll cut back.'
I could try to get a lift.
Maybe I should have a colonoscopy.

I went for a pee and then called Luke back to check in. He didn't answer. Not surprising; he was probably still sorting out the airway, and the phone reception in the unit is notoriously patchy, so I waited another five minutes and texted. Still there was no response, so I put my trousers on.* Then my phone rang and relief washed through me. They'd seen the missed calls and were ringing to tell me to stop worrying.

'Hi,' I said. 'Sorry to keep bothering you. All OK?'

'No.' There was a pause, but I could hear the alarms and raised voices of a medical emergency in the background. 'He's arrested.'

'*Arrested?*' As ever, I failed to keep the emotion out of my voice. 'What happened?'

'We lost the airway.'

'But you've got one now?'

'No.'

'*You haven't got an airway?*'

'Sorry, we're trying. I thought someone had called you.'

By now I had my shoes on and was halfway down the stairs.

'I'm on my way.'

---

* As part of getting dressed. I don't put trousers on as a stress management technique.

'Thanks.'

'Have you got lots of help?'

'Yeah.'

'OK.' I hung up as I left the house and slammed the front door behind me. He sounded terrified and I was starting to regret allowing my own frustration and anxiety to be so obvious in my voice. As I pulled out onto the main road, I called the consultant on call for anaesthetics (I was just on for ICU) just in case she could get there quicker, but she was ten minutes further away than I was.

Halfway in I got stuck at some lights, so I called the registrar again for an update.

'We've got a tube in.'

'Fantastic, well done.'

'But he's still in cardiac arrest.'

'I'll be with you in ten minutes.'

It's strange driving to a medical emergency in your own car. I don't have blue lights or doctor stickers. I don't think I have a legal right to break the law, but it seems wrong to stick to a twenty-miles-an-hour speed limit or sit at an empty pedestrian crossing.

I arrived to an all-too-familiar scene. Fergus was in Bay 3, in the first bed on the right. There's no natural light, but it's a good-sized space that was now filled with trolleys, equipment and noise. Curtains were drawn around the neighbouring beds, but their occupants were awake and would be listening to everything. It was unavoidable. I just hoped it wasn't too frightening for them. Fergus's bed itself was a mess of vials and bloodstained sheets. One staff nurse was leaning over him delivering vigorous chest compressions, while one of the anaesthetists squeezed a bag to ventilate the lungs with one hand and clung to the breathing tube that she'd struggled so hard to insert with the other.

'Two minutes,' someone called. 'Rhythm check and adrenaline, please.'

We all turned to the monitor to look at the heart rhythm, but a depressingly smooth line gently undulated across the screen – asystole. There was no discernible electrical activity passing through Fergus's heart.

'No central pulse,' confirmed an SHO who had one hand dug into Fergus's groin and the other into the side of his neck. There was a heavily bloodstained dressing over the front of his Adam's apple. At some point they'd tried to get into the airway through the front of his neck.

'Back on the chest, please,' the team leader (the post-CCT anaesthetist) requested, and the staff nurse continued her impressive compressions.

'So?' I asked Luke.

'He looked reasonably stable when I first came off the phone so we continued to prepare for intubation. I wanted to get the video laryngoscope and a D-blade, so things took a bit longer than we'd thought and then suddenly he collapsed and desaturated. We tried to bag-mask ventilate him but we couldn't. I think maybe he was in laryngospasm (tight closure of the vocal cords), so we anaesthetized and paralysed him and then tried to intubate, but we couldn't see anything – it was all just horribly swollen with loads of bloodstained secretions and then very quickly he dropped his pressure and arrested. We started CPR and tried again to bag-mask ventilate, tried to intubate twice more, tried a Guedel, LMA, and i-Gel,* then Grace had a go at intubating, but she couldn't see a thing so we tried front-of-the-neck access, but again . . . it was unsuccessful. It was all obviously much more difficult because of the CPR. Eventually Grace got

* A Guedel is a rigid plastic tube that sits along the top of the mouth and ends at the base of the tongue to help keep a patient's airway open. LMA and i-Gel are examples of similar but longer, flexible alternatives that end in the throat above the opening of the larynx. They are also known as supraglottic airways.

a small, six-point-five tube in with a fifth attempt from above. That was fifteen minutes ago – and we've been in asystole ever since.'

It was a remarkably composed description of an appalling sequence of events.

For the next forty minutes we continued CPR. We went through every reversible cause of cardiac arrest (although we were pretty convinced that low oxygen was responsible), we gave multiple rounds of adrenaline, calcium, bicarbonate, fluids and oxygen, but there was no response. We gave a dose of a clot-busting drug, in case this was another heart attack or a massive blood clot to his lungs, but through more than an hour of CPR Fergus's heart did nothing. There wasn't even a flicker of electrical activity. The ventilation delivered oxygen and the chest compressions pushed blood around his body, but his heart showed no signs of coming back to life and then pink frothy secretions started to bubble up through the breathing tube. His lungs were filling with fluid. It was hopeless. Eventually we admitted defeat, and at one thirty in the morning verified Fergus as deceased.

As we trudged out of the bay, the anaesthetic consultant, Caroline, arrived. There was no obligation for her to attend – she knew I was already there – but she appreciated that this was a grim experience for everyone involved. An airway catastrophe – worse, now: an airway death – is every anaesthetist and intensivist's worst nightmare, and the team would need support and a debrief.

I grabbed a glass of water and then went to speak to Fergus's sister, who had just arrived. She'd been called during the CPR and was waiting for me in the relatives' room. She was a slight woman with kind smiling eyes and greying brown hair. She sat still wrapped tight in her knee-length padded black coat.

'Hello,' I began. 'Are you Fergus's sister?'

She looked up at me and I saw the hope fade.

'Yes,' she replied.

'My name is Jim Down, I'm one of the ICU consultants.'

'He's . . . not . . . ?'

'I'm so sorry.'

She looked down and slowly shook her head.

It turned out that she'd been her brother's primary carer. Fergus had had multiple mental as well as physical health problems, and for the last six months they'd been living together. She had been trying to persuade him to go to hospital for days before he'd eventually agreed and she was frustrated as well as heartbroken by his incapacity to look after himself. I was honest about the fact that we had lost control of his airway and I explained that we would do a full review of what had happened and let her know the findings, but she was much more interested in the weeks and months that had led up to this point. While I was obsessing about the final incident that had resulted in Fergus's demise, his sister was thinking about the bigger picture. How had he got to the point of being in ICU on a ventilator again so soon? Perhaps she was feeling guilty about that.

For a while we sat in silence and stared at the wall of bluebells.

'He'd given up on life,' she said. 'Stopped enjoying things, stopped engaging. He just didn't care any more. I tried. I tried to get him out and about, I got the GP in, but Fergus wasn't interested. I guess he'd had enough.' She paused and looked up at me. 'He was a brilliant big brother. Sorry.'

'No, no. Please.'

A tear rolled down her cheek and she began to rifle through her bag for a tissue, so I grabbed some of the NHS hand towels from above the sink and handed her one.

'Thank you,' she said.

Usually it's the other way round. We are trying to get across the bigger picture while the relatives are focused on the single detail that they feel was pivotal, but she was right. Fergus's heart and lungs were not good and his chances of getting out of hospital had already been slim. But that didn't change the fact that we had lost control of his airway.

Twenty minutes later we began a hot debrief.* We spread out around the awkward contours of the ICU seminar room – three registrars, two SHOs, three ICU nurses, Caroline and me, all clasping hot drinks. Occasionally someone advanced to grab a biscuit or a chocolate from the stash in the middle of the room. Only Caroline was emotionally detached from the event. The rest of us had skin in the game. We'd all played some part, from the nurse who'd been looking after Fergus and trying to clear the secretions, to Luke who had spent time assembling extra equipment, to me who had not come in immediately and to the anaesthetists who had struggled to gain control of the airway for over half an hour. We all felt different combinations of shock, fear, doubt and guilt.

As we relived events, it became apparent that the team had followed the national guideline to the letter. Each step they had taken was exactly what the Royal College of Anaesthetists' Difficult Airway Society recommended. Every time a manoeuvre was unsuccessful, they had moved on to the next – and yet still the patient had died. It was only when they had reached the end of the algorithm and made a last-ditch fifth attempt to get the breathing tube in through the mouth (not part of the guidelines) that they were successful – by which time it was too late. What did that mean? One thing it meant was that the team could stand up in any inquest in the country and demonstrate that they were

---

* The aim of a hot debrief is to allow people to talk through what happened from their perspective while it is still fresh in their minds. There are sometimes immediate lessons to be learnt, but the primary purpose is to find out how everyone is feeling and to offer reassurance and support.

beyond reproach, but it also meant that following the guideline does not guarantee a positive outcome.

We all know that; it's obvious. Sticking to the Highway Code does not guarantee that you won't crash your car. Risk can often only be mitigated, not eliminated, but in this case there was another complication to consider.

It is possible that deviating from the algorithm would have led to a favourable outcome. Had they made their attempt to intubate sooner, before trying to get in through the front of the neck, they might have been successful and they might have got the heart started again. Their first four attempts at intubation were in unfavourable circumstances, because the patient was flat on a deflated, low bed with ongoing chest compressions. Intubating anyone in this situation is challenging and Fergus was rotund, with a short, stiff neck, a small mouth, buck teeth and a swollen airway. Four failed attempts was not especially surprising. But the guideline recommends that, rather than try a fifth time, you should move on to other options. If they had deviated from it and the patient had died, an expert witness might have said something like: 'There is a national guideline. It has been put together after careful thought by an erudite panel of experts to avoid just this kind of tunnel vision. Your decision not to follow it is likely to have contributed to this patient's death.'

A fifth attempt at intubation (before going through the front of the neck) would have been looked upon as fixation error – obsession with the task in hand coupled with the inability to pause, think laterally and consider other options. We intubate people every day, almost always successfully, so we can find failure hard to accept. Our field of vision narrows and our ability to think logically is diminished. It is a big step to accept defeat and move on to the far more traumatic and less familiar technique of cutting through the neck, so we can easily push that idea to the back of our minds and kid ourselves that if we just have one more go we'll get the tube in. And then one *more* go after that . . .

This is what the writers of the guideline were worried about. They understood that, under stress, our cognitive ability diminishes and they wanted the options to be ingrained in our consciousness and easily accessible. They didn't want us to be floundering around searching for how and what to do next, they wanted it to be clear and simple and they achieved that. Their document is excellent, but it doesn't tell the whole story – because it can't. The guideline needs to be succinct, but each crisis involves a different patient, a different clinical course, a different time of day and a different group of staff. The guideline can't cover every eventuality and it doesn't explore, for example, the fact that going through the front of the neck might also fail. It doesn't say at the bottom, after front-of-neck access: '– although sometimes this might not work and you might have been better having another go at intubating. Sorry.'

But, as this case demonstrates, you might. In thin people with swan-like necks, finding the windpipe with a scalpel might be easy, but in short, fat people with fixed spines it can be nigh-on impossible. And most of us have never had to try in a life-threatening emergency. We have practised on plastic models and sheep's necks, so we're 'trained', but it's not the same – there is no blood, for a start, or patient's life on the line.

Medical guidelines are a force for good, but they're not infallible. They are not protocols, and we should be cautious both about how slavishly we adhere to them and how we judge those who deviate. Management of an airway emergency is time critical, so the order in which you do things is important. At a certain point it becomes too late. When you make the decision to attempt this or that manoeuvre next, you might be betting a person's life on it. You are making the judgement that in this particular circumstance, for this patient, in your hands, this option has the best chance of success. You are in a place where no one wants to be, the extreme of clinical practice and the 'lost airway' guideline is practical, clear and a great help, but it is a compromise between clarity and reality. There will be circumstances in which sticking to the guideline rigidly results in a life lost that could have been saved. We'll never know which ones because we don't live the counterfactual, just as we'll never know exactly how many lives the guideline has saved. There are no randomized controlled trials and there never will be.

Books have been written about how bad medics are at learning from disasters (in comparison with the airline industry, for example). This might be true, but the books always seem to contain an implied, and in my opinion flawed, assumption. The authors assume that there is a single correct way to do things in medicine, and that doing it will avert disaster. When something goes wrong, they argue, there must have been deficits, be they technical expertise, communication, culture or equipment. Identify and correct those deficits and the problem will be avoided next time. This is wrong. Of course, we should always strive to improve, but we must also acknowledge and embrace the complexity and unpredictability of what we do.

Guidelines, flattened hierarchies and open channels of communication are important, but often in emergencies one person ultimately has to make a tough decision, and quickly. There may be no 'good' option, and luck always plays a part. If the guideline is perceived to be the law then there is the risk of a different form of fixation error – fixation on the algorithm. If we are going to learn, we have to acknowledge all of this and be wary of judgement and heuristics.

In the past, whenever I heard of a case that had ended badly, I used to identify a moment in the narrative when I would have acted slightly differently – just differently enough to have avoided disaster. I did it automatically, inventing my own bespoke guideline for that particular incident that would have got me through. That night I told myself that I'd have demanded CPR stop for as long as I wanted, used a different laryngoscope and insisted upon a further attempt at intubation through the mouth – knowing that front of neck access would have been a nightmare. That way, in my mind, I would have been successful.

In reality, though, I might well not have been, and by deviating from the guideline I would have exposed all of us to criticism. But my trick of the mind served a purpose. It allowed me to carry on. It gave me internal permission to put the next patient to sleep and to site the next tracheostomy. It gave me the confidence to go out there again, a bit like the rituals and superstitions of a sports star before a big match.

Since Covid I've stopped looking for those moments. The scale, brutality and unpredictability of that virus changed something in me that means it doesn't work any more, but it was good while it lasted.

A few years ago I conducted a survey of our anaesthetic department asking which colleague each member would choose to anaesthetize them or their family. (I assumed that people wished their family well, although admittedly I didn't check.) My motivation was to shine a light on the 'unsung clinical stars'. UCH is a London teaching hospital and the plaudits are largely reserved for the academics and medical managers, while there is a tendency to take the outstanding clinicians for granted. I also gave a list of possible reasons for their answers and asked them to score each from most important to least.

The options were:

- Follows latest evidence
- Experience

- Clinical skill/talent
- Knowledge
- Trust
- Judgement
- Professionalism
- Caring/bedside manner
- Attention to detail
- Preference of particular anaesthetic technique
- Management of pain relief
- Performance under pressure/in emergency.

Initially, I added a supplementary question:

- Is there anyone in the department you would actively not want to be anaesthetized by and for what reason?

I asked people not to name names, but then abandoned the supplementary question when there was a minor revolt (although not before a few people had seized the opportunity to make their feelings crystal clear).

Three clinicians stood out as the most popular, and the reasons were plain to see. People valued 'skill/talent', 'knowledge' and 'experience' most highly, in that order. Bottom of the list were 'preference of technique', 'follows latest evidence' and 'caring'. Anaesthetists didn't mind how they were anaesthetized, either technically or personally, and they didn't care if the anaesthetist spent their nights reading or writing pieces for the medical journals. They just wanted the person they thought was best at it. We are all competent, I hope, but some are exceptional, some very good and some just good enough. In stressful circumstances some of us perform better than others. No protocols, guidelines or flowcharts will make us all identical or prevent every catastrophe.

★

The other side of the coin is all the times that I and others have made errors or cut corners, but been lucky and got away with it: the near misses, when we are distracted by one particular aspect of a case and as a result lose sight of another. Derek was a great example. He had a rare and severe heart abnormality and now his bowel had become obstructed by a tumour. He needed to have the tumour removed as an emergency, so I anaesthetized him very carefully, focusing almost entirely on keeping his heart stable. I adapted my technique, checked my drugs and doses far more than was necessary, added more monitoring, managed his fluids and pain relief with precision and booked an ICU bed for afterwards. Derek was also allergic to penicillin, which I sort-of overlooked.

It can feel as if almost everyone is allergic to penicillin. The vast majority of the reactions are minor, often dating back to childhood, but occasionally they're life-threatening anaphylaxis. We have multiple checklists and we quiz patients about their allergies until they are sick of it. Then we make a judgement, asking ourselves: 'Is this just a mild reaction, meaning that we can give an antibiotic related to penicillin that has a 10 per cent rate of crossover allergy, or is it serious enough to avoid anything even remotely similar to penicillin?'

That day, the penicillin allergy was pushed down my priority list by the patient's dodgy heart, the difficult previous case and the family of another patient I was due to meet later, who had made a particularly aggressive complaint. The parking spaces in my brain were filling up, and though I still asked about allergies, I did not give Derek's answer the attention it deserved. He didn't know whether the reaction was severe, because he'd been three years old at the time, but he seemed relaxed about it and the information slipped quickly to the back of my mind. Twenty minutes later I gave the penicillin-related antibiotic. With his heart abnormality, an anaphylactic reaction probably would have killed him.

But he didn't have one, so I got away with it.

I found out later that his reaction to penicillin was severe. Luckily he was *not* part of the 10 per cent who are also allergic to the antibiotic I gave. A shiver went down my spine and I swore I'd be more careful next time. It could have been a fatal mistake and, if it had been, a whole sequence of events would have unfolded. I would have been criticized, investigated and judged – by myself as well as by others. I might then have faced disciplinary proceedings by the GMC and even criminal investigation. But I wasn't, because I was the beneficiary of moral luck.*

Our learning in medicine is driven too much by outcomes and not enough by intention and action. It is human nature to react more strongly to tragic events than near misses, but we should resist the emotional pull and assess every event as dispassionately as possible.

We are told that we work in an open, honest, blame-free culture and are fully accountable to our patients. At first glance that sounds wonderful, but on closer inspection I'm not sure it makes sense, because to be accountable there must be the facility to apportion blame. We can't say, 'I am afraid there has been a screw-up, but no one and nothing is to blame.' It might be an individual, a group of individuals, the institution, the system or a combination of them all, but if there is a 'screw-up' then something must have caused it, and that thing is to blame.

When there is ill-intent, it is easy – someone acting in bad faith obviously needs to be reprimanded – but the vast majority of people go into work with good intentions. They then perform

* Moral luck describes the impact of luck on our moral status. The drunk driver who hits a wheelie bin is an idiot whereas the one who hits a child is a monster – despite the fact that their intention and action may well have been identical. Some philosophers argue that luck has no place in moral status, but in practice we see its place all too clearly every day.

with varying degrees of diligence, compassion, skill and luck, which results in a range of outcomes. If the outcome is unfavourable the diligence, compassion and skill are examined and a judgement is made.

Proof of negligence in any field requires (1) that the defendant has a duty of care to the complainant, (2) that that duty has been breached by a culpable act or omission, (3) that injury has occurred, and (4) that the injury in question is a reasonably foreseeable consequence of the defendant's act or omission. Medical negligence is no different, and the duty of care is taken as read, so it comes down to whether the clinician breached that duty and, if so, was injury caused?

For the last seventy years the test of that breach has been the Bolam Test. John Bolam sustained severe fractures while undergoing electro-convulsive therapy (ECT) in the 1950s. He sought compensation for negligence on the grounds that he was not restrained and he did not receive a muscle relaxant to reduce the risk. He lost his case because 'a responsible body of medical practitioners in the same speciality' said it would have done the same as his doctor. It was not routine to warn people about these risks at the time, nor to use restraint or muscle relaxant. In 1996 the Bolam Test was refined by the Bolitho Test, which clarified that the responsible body's opinion must have a 'logical basis'.

Regarding issues around consent, Bolam and Bolitho have been superseded by the 2015 case of *Montgomery* v. *Lanarkshire Health Board* (see Chapter 11). The ruling of this case stated that patients must be informed in advance about all the material risks of an intervention, whatever the view of the doctor, and recently people have suggested other areas of medical practice for which Bolam is inappropriate. No group of clinicians would make a pure diagnostic error on purpose, so the Bolam Test does not really work in these cases and it doesn't lend itself to situations in which an act, if proved, is agreed by all to be negligent.

I would like to propose a further category for re-examination. What about when clinicians are just a bit crap? When they forget to check something, or get distracted when they are looking at an X-ray, or write a prescription wrong, or bodge a procedure because they are nervous, tired, hungry or sad. And what about when they're paralysed by fear in an emergency, or worried about calling the boss because they think they should be able to do this on their own by now, or give the wrong blood or give the wrong drug or give the right drug by the wrong route – how does a body of your peers deal with that? No body of clinicians could say that they would choose to do any of these things, and yet there are few senior doctors who haven't done most of them at some point in their career. However high the stakes, people cannot be at their very best every day of their working lives, it's not realistic. Everyone makes mistakes. Investigators, coroners, expert witnesses and judges know this, so they take other things into account such as mitigating circumstances, experience, character references, past performance and honour after the event. They mix all of these in with their own preconceptions, biases, emotions and prejudices and try to find the balance between acceptable error and accountability. Within that calculation they have to decide which elements of a clinician's conduct are most important. Is it their level of effort, compassion, knowledge, honesty or skill that matters most? Or is it always the weakest link in the chain? And then, somehow, they have to work out what level of each is acceptable.

Cases with bad outcomes in which concerns are raised about the quality of care are known as 'serious incidents'. I have been lead investigator of several serious incidents at UCH, and each time I have wrestled with these issues. I've always tried to be fair to the clinicians involved and I am acutely aware of hindsight bias, but, if I am honest, I wonder whether I'm too soft on them. I empathize with the doctors. I've been them and I know that they didn't want to cause harm and would do anything to turn back the clock. I've felt the same fear I see in their eyes and sensed their anxiety about how candid to be.

As I anticipated, the internal investigation into Fergus's death concluded that he was managed well. The investigator highlighted a few minor learning points, but felt overall that the team had done an excellent job in challenging circumstances. Nevertheless, everyone involved was upset, and for one registrar in particular the two-month wait for the coroner's inquest was unbearable. We tried to reassure him that there was nothing to worry about, but he couldn't seem to hear us and, looking back, I wonder if we were barking up the wrong tree. Perhaps his reaction wasn't inappropriate. Perhaps we should beat ourselves up more. I wondered how Fergus's sister was getting on.

The coroner agreed with our investigator and returned a verdict of recognized complications of a medical procedure. There is no doubt in my mind that this was the right verdict in this case, but I am still not sure how society should decide where to draw the line.

9.   Death

For me, 2016 was a strange year. Like many, I'd not really taken the threat posed by Brexit or Trump seriously and had been coasting in my comfortable north London bubble, but now suddenly I felt disenfranchised. Politics seemed to be dominated by populism, the climate emergency was slipping down the agenda, and austerity and public sector cutbacks continued. The kids (now aged seven) were doing fine at school and continued to spend most of their free time locked in mortal combat on the kitchen floor, but my mother was starting to exhibit the early signs of dementia – memory lapses and a marked loss of confidence – and Tish and I both felt a new sense of unease about the future. What sort of a world would we be leaving for the children? I was beginning to question things at work as well, aspects of medicine I'd always taken for granted – even the diagnosis and definition of death itself.

Joan was a seventy-three-year-old retired teacher. She was tall, slim and dishevelled, with hair that appeared to have been styled by Boris Johnson. She had a typical combination of smoking-related health conditions: chronic obstructive pulmonary disease (COPD), angina and poor circulation to her legs. After decades of pleading from her husband she'd stopped smoking three years previously, but to a large extent the damage was already done. She'd been in and out of hospital three times in the previous two years, first with a chest infection, then a small stroke and finally a blockage of the artery to her right leg. Each time she'd struggled for a week or so but then rallied and recovered without needing to visit ICU. But these episodes had taken their toll, and since her most recent discharge she'd only got out of the house to make her weekly trip to Sainsbury's via the White Bear pub. But she was still able to care for herself, and her husband, a fashion retailer, continued to work.

Then, on a chilly October afternoon, she fell and fractured her hip. She'd just started a course of antibiotics for a urine infection and stood up too quickly, felt dizzy and collapsed. Her husband discovered her on the kitchen floor when he got home from work an hour later and called an ambulance immediately.

Joan was admitted under the orthopaedic surgeons, given intravenous fluids and more powerful antibiotics overnight and the next morning taken to theatre to have her fractured hip repaired. Initially she did well. She coped with the anaesthetic and was stable when she first came up to the unit afterwards for monitoring, pain relief and antibiotics, but two days later, she developed a sharp pain on the right side of her chest and couldn't catch her breath. Her heart then flicked into an abnormal, fast rhythm, her oxygen levels fell and her blood pressure plummeted. We gave her fluids, put her to sleep, attached her to the ventilator and began infusions of drugs to slow her heart and support her blood pressure.

We then took her for an emergency CT scan of her chest. It confirmed that a large blood clot was blocking one of the major vessels to Joan's lungs (a pulmonary embolus) and a bedside scan of her heart demonstrated that the resulting back pressure was putting her already weak heart under strain. The best treatment option was a clot-busting drug, but her previous stroke and the recent surgery meant that it was high risk. If she bled it could be catastrophic, so I called her husband to explain the situation. I could hear the catch in his voice as he told me to do whatever I thought best and confirmed that he'd come in as quickly as he could.

'I don't drive, unfortunately,' he added. 'So I might be an hour, sorry.'

Having spoken to the surgeon who'd operated on Joan's hip, I decided on balance to give the clot buster and initially it seemed to help. Joan remained dependent on the ventilator, but her heart rhythm settled and her blood pressure stabilized. When her husband arrived (nearly an hour and a half later owing to problems on the Underground) he was clearly distraught, but he put on a brave face and spent the whole day at the bedside, holding his unconscious wife's hand and reminiscing about happier times.

Joan was still stable when I did the evening ward round so I made a plan for the night, updated her husband and suggested he go home and get some rest. We'd call, I reassured him, if anything changed. He thanked us all profusely and begged us to keep trying everything. She was a special lady, he explained, and he wasn't ready to let her go – not yet.

'Of course,' I replied. 'She is in a precarious position, but we're doing everything we can, I promise.'

At 8 a.m. the next day Joan's left pupil dilated and stopped reacting to light. We took her straight down for a CT scan, which showed, as we feared, that she'd bled into her brain. The pressure in her skull was rising and compressing, among other things, the nerves to her left eye. When we got back to the unit I examined her pupils again and discovered that now both left and right pupils were dilated and unresponsive. It was a catastrophic bleed and there was no way back for her now, so I called her husband again. He was just preparing to leave the house, he explained in a flustered voice, and would be there as quickly as he could.

'So please keep trying,' he implored, 'at least until I get there.'

'OK,' I agreed, 'but if it comes to it, we won't do CPR, because I am afraid it would not change the outcome.'

There was a pause on the other end of the line.

'She is essentially already receiving full resuscitation,' I continued. 'If the heart stops despite that, there really is nothing more that we can offer. Doing chest compressions won't restart it. It will just be . . . undignified.'

Cardiopulmonary resuscitation (CPR) is a holding mechanism. It delivers oxygen to the brain, while we try to diagnose and treat the cause of the arrest. The best kind of cardiac arrest to have (in case you are considering one) is ventricular fibrillation – the abnormal heart rhythm that causes it to quiver (fibrillate) rather than beat – because we can deliver an electric shock to a fibrillating heart that might stun the electrical circuits back into a normal, effective rhythm. This is why defibrillators have appeared in train stations, repurposed phone boxes and other public places, but if a heart has stopped and is not in a 'shockable rhythm', the outlook is bleak. The only option is to continue CPR, treat whatever caused the heart to stop beating in the first place and hope that it will start again. If the heart is still not pumping when all the reversible causes have been treated, we stop CPR because it has become futile.

Doctors do not offer treatments that will not benefit their patients. One of the four pillars of medical ethics is beneficence – 'do good' – so if an intervention will not do good then we shouldn't suggest it. This might seem obvious, but it can become complicated. Patients (or their families) sometimes disagree with us about whether a particular treatment could result in a certain outcome and/or whether that outcome represents benefit, because benefit does not necessarily mean cure, or even extended life. It might mean comfort, functional improvement, the ability to leave hospital, or a whole host of other things, but to be considered, a treatment must offer something that is of value to the patient.

But CPR is unique, because the default position is immediate death. Without the CPR the heart is not beating, so for it to be inappropriate the expected result of CPR must be either be death or a fate worse than death. The difficulty is deciding what constitutes a fate worse than death. For most people a certain quality of life (or lack of suffering) is necessary to make it worth living, but for some life itself is sacred and always better than death.

There are broadly three reasons to make patients 'DNR' (do not resuscitate, in full DNACPR – do not attempt cardio-pulmonary resuscitation). The first is that we are convinced that resuscitation will 'almost certainly' be ineffective. In these circumstances CPR can be described as futile because it will not achieve its most basic remit, i.e. to reinstitute the spontaneous circulation of blood. The GMC's guidance for this scenario is that we are not duty bound to inform the patient of the DNR decision, but instead must judge each case on its merits. This is logical because we don't have to tell patients about other futile treatments, so why this one? An ICU patient who is fully investigated, closely monitored and deteriorating despite receiving multiple organ support nicely describes this situation. A patient or relative might ask what 'almost certainly' means, but usually this is fairly clear-cut.

The second circumstance in which we institute a DNR order is when a patient is coming to the end of their natural life – for example, in the final stages of a terminal disease. To die is usually to suffer a cardiac arrest, so to institute a DNR order when someone is known to be dying makes sense. CPR might prolong the process of dying (and rob it of dignity) but it will not add meaningful life. The difficulty in this scenario is deciding when extending life becomes prolonging death. As clinicians we often look grave and nod our heads as we confirm to each other that the patient in front of us is 'dying'. Just saying the words out loud can alleviate the burden of responsibility because the implication is that there is no more we can or should do to extend life. Of course, it is important to be able to accept this, but there is something almost prophetic about the way we say the words – as if we've reached some higher plane of understanding. Do we really always know when people are dying or are we sometimes using our experience to make an educated guess?

As senior trainee intensivists prepare for consultant jobs, they can feel frustrated by the decisions of old codgers like me and sometimes I can sense them rolling their eyes and thinking: 'Why the hell is he still flogging on with this poor old man? He's clearly never getting out of here,' and, 'Why did he admit the woman in Bed 4? She's riddled with metastatic cancer, for Christ's sake.'

The nurses and some of my consultant colleagues sometimes feel the same way, and they may be right. An increasing awareness of my own mortality might be playing a part and sensible decisions have to be made, but my counter is, 'The longer I do the job the more surprises I see.'

None of us is getting out of here alive, but as medicine advances, incurable does not always equate to terminal. People live with cancers for years (decades, sometimes) undergoing a range of life-extending treatments, so identifying the transition from 'living' to 'dying' is not always easy. A sixty-year-old with prostate cancer might never be cured, but he could live with it for years. If he were on a ventilator for an intercurrent pneumonia, his cancer diagnosis would essentially be irrelevant to his CPR status. The metastatic lung cancer (with six-month prognosis) of a forty-six-year-old, on the other hand, is very relevant. Their intercurrent pneumonia is also theoretically reversible, but if they deteriorate to the point of cardiac arrest they will almost certainly need another month on ICU and then probably two more in hospital. These three months will be painful, undignified and exhausting and any planned life-extending cancer treatments will be impossible. They will probably be left with minimal 'quality' time at the end of it, if any, so CPR would almost certainly be prolonging death. The tricky ones, of course, are all the patients who sit somewhere between these two.

The final time we consider a DNR order is when the burdens of the treatment outweigh the benefits. The suffering or indignity of CPR and subsequent life-preserving interventions sometimes dwarfs the possibility of benefit, and the outcome of successful resuscitation may be regarded as worse than death. Should a frail ninety-five-year-old with a fractured hip who suffers a huge blood clot to the lungs be given CPR? The downsides (severe bruising and fractured ribs) probably outweigh the benefits, even in the very few who survive. Should we attempt to resuscitate a patient in a minimally conscious state following a catastrophic head injury? Or someone severely disabled by a stroke or dementia? In each case the period of reduced blood flow during the cardiac arrest will only make the brain function (and thus their quality of life) worse.

The last two categories of DNR orders could be described as 'best interests' decisions. They are based on long-standing ethical principles such as beneficence (do good) and non-maleficence (do no harm), but they can be complex and contentious. Autonomy is the third great ethical pillar, and when a patient has capacity the current position is that they should be involved in the CPR decision. If they disagree with us, the ethical principles may be in conflict and a hierarchy required. Often autonomy is regarded as the central ethical principle, because in a liberal society a person should be allowed to conduct their life in a manner of their choosing. This is borne out when a patient of sound mind refuses any medical intervention (to administer it in those circumstances is assault), but it does not mean that patients will be granted anything they demand (see Chapter 11). Doctors are allowed to withhold all other non-beneficial treatments unilaterally, but, uniquely, we must gain the consent of the patient or next-of-kin to withhold CPR. This has been confirmed by several court cases and raises the question of whether the writing of a DNR form is now regarded as the active medical intervention, rather than the CPR itself – as if CPR is the default and to write a DNR form is to deviate from 'normal life expectations'. Perhaps a better description is that we are deciding between two different medical interventions and so either choice requires consent. It remains an odd situation, though, because currently there is more onus on us to get consent *not* to perform CPR than to do it. I don't know of any other medical intervention where that is the case.

Do I think that CPR should be viewed as different from other treatments and conferred special status? On balance, I don't. I do believe that it is an unusual intervention, so warrants discussion more often than others, but mandating that we always talk about it probably causes more harm than good. That might sound patronizing, but when a patient is dying it often feels insensitive and unnecessary to burden them with a conversation about the inappropriateness of chest compressions. Some of you may be relieved to hear, however, that it doesn't matter what I think, because the national guidance disagrees. The GMC position is that unless we are convinced that CPR will 'almost certainly' not lead to the return of a spontaneous circulation, or that the discussion will cause physical or psychological harm to the patient, then we should always include them in a DNR decision.

There is also the other side of the coin. Should we assume that people want to be given CPR when we think they'll benefit or should we double check with every patient as they arrive in the hospital?

'Good morning, Johnny, how did your A levels go? All set for your toenail removal? Good! Oh, by the way, if your heart stops, do you want us to try to restart it?'

'*What?*'

'I'm sure it'll be fine, but –'

'Why are you asking me that?'

'Well, you know – cover all the bases.'

'*Mummm!*'

Death is something that people like Johnny have often barely considered, and certainly would rather not think about, and this conversation is unlikely to improve their patient experience. Naturally, there are ways to reduce the distress, but do I ask every eighteen-year-old coming for minor surgery whether they want CPR? No, I don't. I take the view that the psychological harm of bringing up the subject outweighs the tiny chance that a healthy eighteen-year-old will both suffer a cardiac arrest and also not want CPR. By the letter of the law I probably should check, but I'll take that risk.

To start CPR on Joan would have been illogical for two reasons. Firstly, we were convinced that she couldn't make a meaningful recovery from her current predicament and, secondly, we felt that if she went into cardiac arrest we'd not be able to restart her heart.

'OK,' Joan's husband replied to my statement about CPR, 'but please keep supporting her until I get there. I am bringing someone – a friend.'

There was something slightly odd about the way he said 'friend', but I didn't want to put him or his friend off coming so I didn't question it.

'Absolutely,' I agreed. 'Good idea, and we'll keep doing what we are doing, but, as I say, if her heart stops –'

'Yes, I know.'

Half an hour later, despite our support, Joan passed away. The rising pressure in her brain caused her blood pressure to soar and then her heart to slow dramatically. A few minutes after that, as the pauses between heartbeats lengthened, the oxygen levels and blood pressure fell and soon both faded away to nothing. We verified her death in the normal way, checking for a pulse, heart sounds, pupil reaction etc. and then waited. Forty-five minutes later her husband arrived with a short middle-aged woman in jeans and a thick cardigan, so I took them both, along with Joan's ICU nurse, Jenny, to the relatives' room.

'I am so sorry,' I began. Then I looked up. Joan's husband glanced anxiously across to his companion. She took his hand but continued to hold my gaze, unmoved, so I continued, 'but I am afraid Joan passed away about forty-five minutes ago. As I said before, the bleed in her brain was catastrophic and the subsequent rise in pressure in her head put strain on her already weak heart. After that, despite our support, her blood pressure soon faded away and then her heart stopped.'

Joan's husband bowed his head for a moment and then looked again at his friend, who nodded.

I waited.

'Thank you,' the woman said. 'I'd like to go in . . . and see her. Is that OK?'

Relatives often ask to spend some time with the deceased, but something felt wrong.

'Yes,' I replied, 'If Mr . . . ?'

'Yes, please,' Joan's husband confirmed.

'We understand what you've said and we appreciate all that you've done,' the woman added calmly, 'but I'd like to try . . . to bring her back.'

'I'm sorry . . . ?'

'I know there's nothing more you can do, but I've been in this situation before.'

'Umm.' I looked over at Jenny, but she was studiously avoiding eye contact.

'And I think I can make her better.'

'She has been dead for nearly an hour,' I repeated. 'There is no way she can be resuscitated now.'

'As I said, I fully understand there's nothing more *you* can do, but I would like to spend some time with her, if you don't object?'

'Well . . .'

'Half an hour.'

I can still picture myself sitting there, completely stunned. On the one hand, I didn't want to upset Joan's husband by denying his wishes, but on the other . . .

'OK,' I said.

I like to think I was being magnanimous and open minded, but it is just as likely I was being cowardly and avoiding conflict.

'If you are happy, Jenny?'

'Um, yeah, fine,' Jenny stammered, looking as if she didn't know whether to laugh or cry.

As I drew the curtains around Joan, her husband and their 'friend' I glanced at the other patients. She was in Bed 20 in the middle of Bay 2, surrounded by four others, two of whom had visitors. What would they make of what was about to happen behind Joan's curtains? Then I was hit by a wave of doubt. What if we'd missed a weak pulse, she wasn't dead and they pulled back the curtains ten minutes later, triumphant. We've all read stories about people waking up in mortuaries.

I spent the next half hour on edge. I left the bay and tried to get on with the rest of the day's work, but my mind kept drifting back to what might be going on behind the curtains of Bed 20.

Joan has been dead for an hour, I kept reminding myself. *She has been washed and laid out by trained nurses. She is not going to rise again.*

Eventually, Joan's husband and his friend emerged. He took my hand and nodded. He was too upset to speak, but his friend smiled warmly, and thanked me. Then she took his hand and off they went. This time she had not been able to raise the dead, but she seemed unperturbed. You win some, you lose some, I suppose.

I have always struggled with DNR orders and other decisions around dying, but I thought that death itself was straightforward. I considered it an objective phenomenon. You were either dead or not. Humans have been dying since they walked the earth, and while medical advances might delay the inevitable, we always lose in the end. I didn't question the criteria that I had dutifully learnt at medical school for confirming or 'verifying' death and I wrote people off who did as crackpots or religious fanatics. I'd spent sleepless nights worrying about what might happen after death (probably nothing, I'd reluctantly concluded) but the concrete reality of the event was beyond debate.

I found Joan's friend amusing (once she had failed). I told a version of the story as an anecdote to colleagues, arrogant in my medical superiority. I was following the science, sticking to established guidelines. When the heart stopped for five minutes or the brain stem no longer functioned, the patient was dead – there was no debate. Our criteria were solid and any other narrative was either twaddle or theoretical philosophy with no practical application. But now I'm not so sure. I still think the criteria are good, but they're not definitive, and death is a much more slippery concept than I'd blithely assumed.

I haven't gone maverick, I don't run around the hospital attempting to raise people who have been certified dead, but I have concluded that death is a process, not a moment, and that the set of parameters we have chosen to define it are a compromise. It is also context specific, and I think it is highly likely that in a hundred years' time we will manage and define death very differently.

Doctors only became involved in verifying death during the eighteenth century. Before that it was largely the domain of the clergy and the immediate family, but the advent of cardiopulmonary resuscitation and the fear of being buried alive (scratch marks were discovered on the inside of coffins) led to the desire for a more robust process. The diagnosis of death needed to be safe (to avoid inadvertent live burial) and timely (to avoid the need to keep putrefying bodies waiting in unrefrigerated mortuaries for days – 'just to be sure' – before burying them). The problem was that the more timely the process, the less safe and vice versa.

The father of modern death diagnosis was Eugène Bouchut, a French physician, who in 1846 won the Paris Academy of Sciences' competition to establish a 'safe, prompt and easy' method to verify people as deceased. He suggested the use of a stethoscope to establish the absence of a heartbeat for five minutes.[*] Nearly two centuries later, verification of death by cardiac arrest is still carried out in a similar way. Junior doctors faithfully listen for a heartbeat and feel for a pulse for five minutes. They also check that the pupils do not react to light and that there is no response to painful stimuli to confirm irreversible loss of consciousness. They then note down the time and document that the patient has died.

In my first few years as a junior doctor I verified the death of dozens of patients (not a suspiciously high number – just to be clear) and there was never any doubt in my mind that they were

---

[*] Other entries to the competition included assessing for any response to leeches placed around the anus and to vices attached to the nipples, so it is safe to say that the standard was not universally high.

dead. I remember the first one vividly. It was the first time I had seen a dead body in the hospital and it was a shock, but it wasn't difficult or stressful. It seemed a bit odd that the time of death was documented as the time of my examination, when clearly it had actually occurred earlier, but there was nothing we could do about that. We couldn't always be there at the moment of death (that *would* start to look suspicious), and a safe medical confirmation seemed more important than getting the time exactly right. Now I have come to the conclusion that there never really was a moment.

Over the years, several august bodies have made attempts to define death, and in 2008 the code of practice of the Academy of Medical Colleges described it as follows:

> Death entails the irreversible loss of those essential characteristics that are necessary to the existence of a living human person, and thus the definition of death should be regarded as the irreversible loss of the capacity for consciousness combined with the irreversible loss of the capacity to breathe. This may be due to a wide range of problems in the body for example cardiac arrest.

In essence what they are saying is that either the heart stops, leading to death of the brain (here defined as the irreversible loss of the capacity for consciousness and to breathe), which is known as death by cardiac arrest, or the brain dies from another cause in the presence of a beating heart, known in the UK as brain-stem death.

This definition is practical and pragmatic, but it does beg questions about both cardiac and brain-stem death.

To examine death from cardiac arrest first, imagine two eighty-five-year-old friends, Sally and Bridget, who ended up in hospital, one on the fourth floor and one on the fifth. They were both previously fit and living full lives, but on New Year's

Day both slipped on a patch of ice, fell and broke their hips (stick with me). They both consented to surgery and were then asked whether they would like CPR in the event of a cardiac arrest. Sally said she'd like everything as long as there was a chance that she might recover, because she was determined to make it to her granddaughter's wedding in four months, but Bridget said no thank you.

'If my heart stops,' she proclaimed, 'for goodness' sake do not jump up and down on my chest. Just let me go peacefully.'

Each decision seemed reasonable and the medical teams dutifully signed Sally as for CPR and Bridget as DNR. The system was working well.

Their operations went smoothly, but three days later at 10.30 a.m., both women suffered huge heart attacks and went into cardiac arrest (I know, but hang in there). Sally's cardiac arrest on the fourth floor was witnessed by a first-year student nurse who pressed the emergency buzzer, but did not feel confident to start CPR. The cardiac-arrest team arrived five minutes later and started CPR. Upstairs, Bridget's cardiac arrest was witnessed by a junior doctor, who, knowing that she was not for CPR, listened for heart sounds and felt for a pulse for five minutes and then verified her as dead and went to call her relatives. Forty minutes later, Sally's heart had not restarted so the cardiac arrest team called a halt to the CPR.

At the five-minute point, just before the cardiac arrest team reached Sally, the two women's physiological status was identical and yet Bridget was defined as dead and Sally alive. This is because CPR is defined as prolongation of life, not resurrection from the dead. If the cardiac arrest team had taken another minute (or even five minutes) to arrive, the two women's physiology would have continued to be identical and yet Bridget would, of course, still have been dead and Sally alive.

This story illustrates that death, though ultimately real, is a process around which we have constructed definitions, just as Bouchut did in 1846. These definitions are context sensitive and need to be re-evaluated as medical practice and societal values change. The fact that death exists does not mean that the point of transition from life to death is either known or set in stone (as it were).*

The concept of brain-stem death (or total brain death, as it is labelled in the USA) arose from our ability to ventilate people artificially for prolonged periods in ICU. This led to situations in which a ventilated person's brain could stop functioning while their heart continued to beat. The brain (in particular the lower part, the brain stem) is required to drive a person's breathing, but if supplied with oxygen, nutrients and a favourable milieu the heart can continue to beat independently. Not only that, with good ICU care the kidneys, liver, gut and immune system may also continue to function and there are case reports

---

* The Academy of Royal Colleges description of death cited above uses the word irreversible three times. If we apply this to the cases of Bridget and Sally, then at the five-minute mark, either both are dead or both alive. If Sally's situation is still potentially reversible then so is Bridget's, so to declare one dead and the other not is illogical. We have added what is 'appropriate' to our thinking alongside what is physiologically possible. To be physiologically consistent it would be better to say that both had died at five minutes and that the CPR is an attempt to bring Sally back to life, but the word irreversible is chosen specifically to avoid that. If we added treating the deceased to our remit it might start to look like a very different job. A better solution might be to replace the word 'irreversible' with 'permanent'. Bridget's heart has stopped permanently at five minutes, even if not strictly irreversibly. It *will* not restart, but that does not mean it *could* not.

But even the word permanent has problems, because if we decide that a cardiac arrest is permanent and so stop CPR then it will *become* permanent. Our decision to stop is a judgement, informed by knowledge and experience, but still a judgement not a fact.

of brain-stem-dead patients who are pregnant successfully gestating their foetuses to term.

UK law mandates that two experienced clinicians follow a strict protocol to confirm brain-stem death and then repeat it to be absolutely sure. Crucially, the final test of the protocol involves disconnecting the patient from the ventilator for five minutes to check for any signs of breathing. More than once I have been convinced that a patient is brain-stem dead only to be proved wrong by a huge intake of breath two minutes into this test. If the patient takes no breath, however, and the other tests reveal no signs of brain-stem activity, the patient is verified dead. They may look very much alive on the ventilator, with a strong pulse and a healthy complexion, but legally they have died.

Relatives often struggle to accept this and do not want us to turn off the ventilator, so we are flexible (within reason). We allow the family time to say goodbye and we give them the opportunity to consider organ donation, but after that we turn off the machines. The time of death is recorded as the time at which the first set of brain-stem death tests was completed.

Until 2016 I had never questioned this. Patients with catastrophic brain injury who did *not* meet brain-stem death criteria were difficult, because their outlook, though probably awful, was still unclear. Determining prognosis and best interests for them was beset with problems, but the patients whose brains had died were straightforward. The only challenge was to persuade the families of the tragic but incontrovertible truth.

We could have defined brain death differently. We might have decided that someone in a persistent vegetative state (PVS), whose brain stem is still functioning, has legally died. By definition they have no psychologically interpretable contact with their environment so, if to be alive and have personhood you need to be aware and interact, then PVS patients are not alive. Often we make judgements about the value of such lives and limit the treatments we offer, such as ventilatory support, admission to hospital or even antibiotics. If their life is of so little worth that it does not merit the use of antibiotics, then is it really a life at all? We would have to establish a different set of criteria to define death, but, having done so, we could stop expensive interventions, enact dignified ends and potentially save extra other lives by organ donation.

Defining PVS patients as dead has practical, ethical, cultural and philosophical difficulties that preclude it from gaining widespread acceptance in the current climate. Safety would be a grave concern. Studies have demonstrated that up to a third of patients with minimally conscious state (MCS, a syndrome in which there is some limited perception of environment) are misdiagnosed as PVS. New technologies such as functional MRI, which show areas of the brain lighting up in response to certain words and stimuli, have added to the controversy, and even if accurately diagnosed, prognosticating about patients in low consciousness states is notoriously difficult. And why draw the line there? What about patients with end-stage dementia, or babies born with very limited brain function?

Many people define consciousness as 'awareness of one's environment', so we could use this as the cut-off. If you are permanently unaware of your environment, then it might be argued that as a person you have died, but in medicine there is general consensus that consciousness comprises both awareness and arousal. PVS patients may not be aware, but they do show signs of arousal or wakefulness (and sleep cycles) because these are controlled by the brain stem. The medical profession therefore considers them to be conscious, and so potentially capable of personhood, and thus alive.

The other objection to our current brain-stem death definition is the reverse. Does the fact that a person fulfils the brain-stem death criteria guarantee that they have died? Assuming that we view the brain and not the rest of the body as the essence of a person (another whole philosophical debate), then the question boils down to whether our criteria definitively describe a brain that has died, i.e. lost the potential for consciousness and respiration.

One reason to doubt (or at least have anxiety about) this is that different countries define brain death in different ways. The USA demands total brain failure,* while in the UK clinical tests that indicate loss of the 'integrative functions of the brain stem (including loss of breathing)' suffice. In some European countries supplementary tests, such as electro encephalograms (EEGs: measurement of electrical activity within the brain) are required, in others the supplementary tests are mandated only under certain circumstances and some countries do not require the test for lack of breathing.

There have been many calls for an international standard, but at the time of writing it is still possible to be legally dead in one country and yet alive in another. Why? Because, again, in trying to find a balance between safety and practicality different countries have drawn the line in different places.

So is it possible to be diagnosed as brain-stem dead in the UK and yet still retain (or regain) consciousness? Theoretically, yes. It is vanishingly unlikely, and in the vast majority of cases can be ruled out categorically, but it is anatomically possible that a lesion could destroy all the areas examined in the brain-stem death tests, but leave consciousness intact.

That would mean that some people (with very specific lesions) whose tests indicate brain-stem death might actually be aware and suffering from total locked-in syndrome. They could have fixed dilated pupils, be unable to blink, breathe,

---

* Strictly speaking, this means no brain function at all, although this is not adhered to because the brain produces hormones and the Americans do not insist that it stops doing that to be declared dead.

move their eyes, cough or gag, and yet still be aware. That might seem like a tortured state to be in, but many people with less complete locked-in syndrome (who can only blink, for instance) describe their lives as full and valuable. With technological advances, particularly brain–computer interfaces, the potential for both communication and even movement for these patients is improving all the time.

Some argue that people with certain lesions causing brain-stem death should, therefore, undergo ancillary tests to rule out higher electrical activity (and thus consciousness), but no consensus has been reached. Those against further testing maintain that it is unnecessary because there has never been a documented case of recovery following the diagnosis of brain-stem death and that the added tests will yield inconclusive and inaccurate results.

My own view is that our current criteria are excellent, but we have not, as I had previously thought, sorted it all out. Just as this is not the end of history, so it is not the end of science or philosophy, and debate must continue. Why, for example, do we set so much store on the ability to breathe when we can so easily support it? We do so because it is easy to test and is a sensitive marker of brain-stem function, but is it so important to the essence of being alive? If consciousness is the key component of life, then perhaps our struggle to determine when a life has ended should focus on that. The brain stem is crucial because it controls arousal, a component of consciousness, but the other component, awareness, is controlled by the higher centres, which we do not test.

We must not lose sight of the fact that diagnosing death needs to be universal, safe, timely and practical. This is as true today as it was when Bouchut was trying to define it. The protocol for brain-stem death in the UK scores well on all those fronts, but in the next few years it might be time to re-examine ancillary testing in certain circumstances. It would also help if we could agree a global definition.

I now feel slightly ashamed that I was so scornful of the 'friend' who came to revive Joan. I have led countless prolonged unsuccessful resuscitation attempts. Are they really so different? It is easy to be dismissive of unfamiliar practices while blithely assuming that everything we do makes perfect sense. We see it every day in the worlds of religion and politics and sometimes in medicine. I liked to think that my approach to death and dying was consistent, rational and logical, but it wasn't. Compassion, guilt, fear, ignorance, insecurity and exhaustion affect my attitude and decision making at work, just as they do in every other aspect of my life. I am grateful for the guidelines and laws in this country that protect both patients and clinicians, but neither I nor the system is perfect. I'm not saying that I think the friend was on to something, or that we should give every madcap opinion the oxygen of publicity, but I still think of her whenever I stand beside Bed 20 on the unit. I believe wholeheartedly in the scientific approach of Western medicine, but I also think that extraordinary advances must be matched by humble acceptance of all that we still do not know or understand.

10. Trust

'How do you learn to break bad news?'

Over the first ten years of my career I was asked that question many times by non-medical friends and each time it put me on edge, because I wasn't quite sure of the answer.

How did I acquire the skills to deliver the worst news that the person in front of me would ever receive? What was the training for managing the conversation that would change their life for ever; for dealing with the moment that they and their family would never forget?

There was certainly no module at medical school or section in my postgraduate exams about communication and empathy. There was a lot about the physics of MRI scanners and different techniques for measuring pressure and humidity (anaesthetic exams are particularly nerdy), but there were no multiple-choice questions about how best to gain a family's trust or to pick up on subtle signals of distress, or about how much time to leave between sentences when delivering complicated and unwelcome medical information.

'It's a sort of apprenticeship,' I usually mumbled in response. 'You watch your various bosses and then try to remember the good bits of each. Gradually you develop a style that works for you and then you stick with it.'

I can see the obvious flaw in my logic.

'A style that works for *you*?'

Surely it should have been a style (if style is even the appropriate word) that worked for the patients and their relatives. Perhaps that's what I meant by 'works for you', but the mere fact that I wasn't sure did not bode well. How carefully and skilfully we treat a person at the most vulnerable time of their life might not alter their prognosis, but it can transform their experience and furnish their family with a completely different set of memories.

I'd tagged along with my bosses to many 'difficult conversations' and I'd been astonished by the range of approaches and by the reactions of both patients and families. I'll never forget the day that my consultant informed a family that their elderly, artist mother was dying, to be met with the reply, 'Thank you, Doctor, we understand. But do you mind if we bring one last therapist in to see her. We don't want to be a nuisance but Mum has been seeing this guy for years, he works with crystals and –'

'Listen,' my boss interrupted, 'you can hang a dead pigeon round her neck as far as I am concerned, it's not going to change the outcome.'

I braced myself for the inevitable gasps of horror and could already see the letters of complaint in my mind's eye, but the family saw the mischievous but kind smile on the consultant's face and smiled back.

'Thank you, Doctor, you've been very clear.'

Even back then I was self-aware enough to realize that the dead pigeon line would not work in my hands, but I assumed that as long as I was kind and caring, I'd be fine.

I didn't receive sackfuls of complaints, so I was probably adequate, but as I settled into my consultant job I focused on the process more and more, and by 2018 I had developed a routine.

These days I take a second person with me, be it the patient's specialist, a trainee doctor or a nurse (and sometimes all three). I introduce myself, ensure that I know who everyone in the room is and then ask the relatives or patient to tell me what they understand of the situation. That gives me an idea of how they are feeling and coping and also ensures that I don't repeat things, miss out a crucial piece of information or contradict one of my colleagues.* Allowing the family to speak first also gives me insight into their level of medical knowledge. It is not ideal to talk to a professor of haematology about the blood being a bit sticky, but I've done it – more than once.

Then I gradually build on the story they have started, filling in the blanks and explaining each step. I have wondered in the past whether I should stop being so long-winded and cut to the chase, but telling the story clarifies how we've reached our painful conclusion and builds trust. It also removes niggling doubts and questions that can otherwise plague relatives for years.† Having delivered the bad news, I pause. It can be disturbing to witness the devastating impact of your words on a relative stranger, and the more I do it (or, perhaps, the older I get), the more emotional I find it.

My first sensation is often a spike of anxiety.

Is there really no hope? Should I have done one more test?

And then guilt.

I could have done that better – been more gentle and used different language.

The balance between being clear and softening the blow must be finely judged, and the urge to sugar-coat the information and

---

* That's not a cover-up. I'm talking about differences of communication style rather than of medical facts. A previous doctor may have used the word 'tumour' instead of 'cancer' or 'sedated' rather than 'asleep', and concordance of terminology minimizes confusion and anguish.

† Having placed my mother in a nursing home under Covid restrictions, I now appreciate how unnerving it is to hand over the care of a loved one to complete strangers. Questions flick through your mind all the time, such as 'Does he really know that she had a good breakfast, or is he busy and just trying to get me off the phone?' I didn't mind people saying, 'I'm not sure. I will just find out for you,' but I hated it when I suspected they were making things up.

downgrade the negatives by using euphemisms can be over-whelming. Replacing words like 'cancer' with 'growth', and 'dying' with 'deteriorating despite our best efforts', can make the news feel less shocking, and that can be helpful – as long as the information is still clear and understood. But many people cling to the possibility of a positive outcome, so we have to be mindful of blurring the message and giving them false hope.

Often the more difficult conversations are when the situation is not clear-cut: when the patient is in a very difficult but not hopeless situation or when they might have the potential to recover, but only after months of painful rehab and only to a dependent state. To say 'What do you think they would want in this terrible situation?' can open up a discussion fraught with hazard, but we have to ask the family this question, because the patient may have expressed strong views (most people haven't). What we don't want to do is leave the relatives with the feeling that 'pulling the plug' on their loved one is their responsibility. Ultimately the decision to withdraw or withhold therapy is a medical one, but it's also one that we always make in consult-ation with the next of kin.

It can take time, but in the vast majority of cases we reach agreement eventually. Occasionally a second opinion is required and the family can, of course, challenge our decision through the courts, but that is still extremely rare.

Sometimes however, despite our best efforts, these 'breaking bad news' conversations do not go to plan.

Carla was a slight, fifty-one-year-old woman, originally from Mexico. She came to the United Kingdom to study architecture, met an English man and never left. They had two children, aged nine and six, and both worked for large London firms. In 2018 Carla presented to UCH Emergency Department with severe necrotic pancreatitis secondary to gallstones. Within a few days her organs were beginning to shut down, she'd developed signs of a chest infection and on day six she needed ventilation. Four days after that she was still getting worse, so the gastroenterologists decided to remove the driver of the pancreatitis by clearing out the gallstones from her bile duct via an endoscopy. During that procedure they noticed some suspicious-looking tissue around the bile duct, so they took biopsies. It was probably all reactive inflammation from the pancreatitis, they thought, but they couldn't be sure. Over the next few days, Carla settled into the long, grim course of a patient with severe pancreatitis, but unlike my friend Sean (see Chapter 6), her lungs were also inflamed. She clearly wouldn't be getting off the ventilator anytime soon, so we inserted a tracheostomy. That same evening the biopsy results came back and our worst fears were realized. Not only did Carla have severe pancreatitis, she also had pancreatic cancer – indeed, the cancer had probably driven the inflammation. The radiologists looked at her CT scan with this new information and confirmed that Carla's cancer was not operable. Even if she'd been otherwise well, she'd only have had a few months to live.

She was still sedated when we received this information, so we called in her family to tell them the bad news. I ushered Carla's husband, mother and brother-in-law into the relatives' room along with her gastroenterologist and the bedside nurse, closed the door and perched, as ever, on the bin. My colleague did most of the talking.

As we recapped the story, the family sat on the edges of their seats, nodding in response to everything we said with the fixed, slightly desperate smiles that we see so often on the faces of ICU relatives. Finally, we got to the nub of the conversation.

'As you know,' the gastroenterologist continued, 'we also sent some samples to the lab.' He looked up at Carla's husband. 'The results came back today.'

I saw the panic in her husband's eyes as they flitted back and forth between my colleague and me.

'Unfortunately,' he continued slowly, 'it is not good news. I am so sorry.' He paused to let the information sink in.

Carla's husband sat motionless. His jaw was tight and his eyes like saucers as he fought back the tears. His brother put a comforting arm around his shoulders. Carla's mother stood up and looked skittishly at all the faces around the room, as if someone else might give her different news.

'What does it mean, not good news?' she asked, clutching the surgeon's arm.

'As well as the inflammatory cells we'd expect from pancreatitis, the pathologists can see cancer cells,' he told her.

'*Cancer?*'

'I am so sorry. I did mention that we had taken biopsies, but I didn't expect –'

'So what now?'

My colleague took a deep breath.

'We've looked back at the scans and I am afraid –'

'*No!*' Carla's mother interjected.

'I am afraid that the tumour has spread too far to be removed.'

'Chemotherapy?'

My colleague looked over at me.

'She's not strong enough to have chemotherapy,' I said.

The six of us sat in silence for a minute.

'So, how long?' her husband asked.

'I don't know,' the gastroenterologist replied. 'Unfortunately pancreatic cancer –'

'Don't tell her,' her mother said suddenly. 'Please don't tell her, she'll give up hope.'

'She's not awake enough for us to talk to her at the moment,' I confirmed, 'so we won't say anything now, but –'

'Thank you,' her mother interrupted again. 'She needs hope.

What good will it do, telling her? She needs to keep fighting – for her children.'

The conversation ended shortly after that and, at their insistence, I promised not to tell Carla until we had talked again.

We woke Carla up gradually over the next few days, but she was getting no closer to escaping the ventilator. We removed every obstacle we could, but each time we reduced her support she became breathless and distressed. Her daughters came in to visit and even climbed onto the bed to hug her, but as time went by I felt increasingly uncomfortable. We should tell her the results. If she had asked, I would have been honest, but she didn't. The gastroenterologist felt that we could reasonably wait a bit longer and try to get her off the ventilator first, but I disagreed. Our duty of care was to Carla. She was going through days of difficult, painful treatments without the prospect of a cure and I felt that she had the right to know her prognosis. She might decide that she'd had enough and ask us to shift our focus and allow nature to take its course. We couldn't conjure up a happy ending. It was a devastating situation, but by keeping quiet we were putting her through miserable treatments on false pretences. She might be hating every second of her existence, but clinging to the hope that, if she just kept fighting, she'd get better.

And she was definitely a fighter. She didn't want to be sedated, she wanted to be awake and exercising, to build up her strength. She smiled warmly when I arrived to examine her each day and nodded determinedly when I asked if she was OK.

It took us another five days, but eventually we persuaded her relatives and told Carla the diagnosis. She accepted the news bravely. Perhaps she had her suspicions already or perhaps she was just exhausted, but there was no grand show of emotion, just a nod of quiet acceptance and hugs for all her family. We all agreed that we'd keep her on ICU, but that if she deteriorated, we wouldn't increase her level of artificial support. A few days later she developed another chest infection and passed away peacefully in her sleep with her husband at the bedside. Her family thanked us for looking after her.

We could have gone against their wishes and told her the diagnosis sooner, but in retrospect I am glad that we didn't. They already had their grief to deal with, and the challenge of raising two children without a mother. I am pleased that we avoided the extra burden of conflict, but ultimately our duty of care was to Carla, so if we had not been able to persuade her family when we did, I would have told her. But I would have hated doing it.

I'd always thought that when relatives wanted us to keep information from patients they were well-meaning, but misguided. More recently, however, I'm less sure that total honesty always passes the 'what I would want' test. If a patient does not want to know every lurid detail about their situation, then as long as it doesn't push us down an unethical treatment path, I do my best to respect their wishes. One could argue that we're all avoiding truths about our own health by not having a full-body CT scan and set of blood tests every year. As a GP friend once said to me, 'Good health is merely a state of inadequate medical investigation.'

But to live, we have to accept an element of uncertainty, and where to draw the line should, when possible, be decided by the individual. If a person wants to ignore the lump growing on the side of their leg, then surely that is their prerogative. In a study of Polish medical students 93 per cent of them felt that their patients should always be told their terminal diagnosis, but only 86 per cent would want to know if they were dying. Each situation is unique and requires a careful, bespoke approach. Most importantly, we mustn't stop listening to the patients.

But occasionally a patient and their family's determination not to engage with their situation makes ongoing management very difficult.

Sonia was in her early forties and suffering with refractory leukaemia. She had undergone two bone-marrow transplants, but her type of blood cancer was particularly aggressive and had returned after both. Cure was no longer possible and, just as palliative options were being discussed, she developed pneumonia and ended up in ICU. When we drained some fluid from around her infected lung we discovered that it was packed with cancer cells, so now her outlook was even more bleak. She only had a few weeks to live, but she responded to the antibiotics and improved enough to be weaned off the ventilator. All of us agreed, however, that having taken the breathing tube out, we should not put it back in, because we'd never get her off the ventilator a second time, so I called in her sister and husband to discuss the plan.

They were grateful for the update but irrepressibly optimistic – confident that God would look after Sonia. The haematologists had already told them about her prognosis, but they didn't seem to understand the gravity of the situation so I tried to clarify.

'I hope she will breathe well,' I said, 'and that we will get her off the ICU, and even home, but there is a good chance that she will deteriorate again, and if that happens –'

'We don't want to think about that,' her husband interjected.

'OK,' I replied, 'I understand, but we have to plan for all potential outcomes and –'

'You mustn't give up on her.'

I took a deep breath. 'I'm not –'

'Miracles happen. She can get better. I know she can.'

'But –'

'She can do this. You just need to support her.'

Sonia was officially still for CPR in the event of a cardiac arrest and I couldn't change that without discussing it with her next of kin, so I tried again.

'We will focus, of course, on getting her better, but if . . . say her heart stopped, I don't think it would be right to do CPR.'

'We do not agree to that.'

'Because?'

'She can get through this.'

'And we'll support her. We'll do everything that might help her.'

'Including CPR?'

'All right,' I conceded, 'I won't make her DNR now –'

'Thank you, Doctor; thank you for everything you are all doing.'

'No problem. We'll speak very soon.'

I had two subsequent meetings with Sonia's family, and I left all three feeling that I had failed. There was now no ambiguity: the situation was black and white. This poor woman was going to die within the next three weeks whatever we did, and yet I couldn't convey that to the family.

For forty-eight hours Sonia was awake and quite comfortable. I tried to talk to her about CPR, but she too did not want to engage. Her extended family all visited and she talked to them lucidly and laughed and hugged her son, but on the third day she inevitably began to tire. Her breathing became increasingly shallow, and as the carbon dioxide built up in her blood, she became drowsy and then gradually unconscious.

My stint on the unit came to an end and I handed over to a colleague feeling slightly embarrassed and guilty. Sonia was in the illogical position of being still for CPR, but not for re-ventilation. If her heart stopped, we'd almost certainly not get it started again, but if by a miracle we did, then she'd definitely need ventilation to keep it going – which we were not offering. I claimed it was a compromise, to avoid excessive futile interventions, while also minimizing further upset and conflict. Or was I being a coward? Perhaps I should have taken a harder line and insisted on a DNR order because my duty of care was to the patient and CPR was not in her best interest. I don't like conflict and I may have been worn down over the years by the desperation of families facing such grim circumstances, but I justify my actions with the 'hierarchy of feelings'. Everyone involved felt upset or frustrated or angry, but it was Sonia's life, so she was the top priority, the relatives would remember these moments for ever, so they should be left with as few doubts and regrets as possible, and the nurses would be at her bedside throughout. I might take ultimate responsibility, but I was not living it like they all were, so my feelings were the least important. (This sounds obvious, but when emotions are running high or plans become controversial it's something that can easily be forgotten.) I didn't think CPR would help Sonia, but neither did I think it would cause undue suffering. It might look painful and undignified, and it might not be the way I'd choose to die, but we could ensure that she was unaware throughout. I felt that leaving her for CPR was a reasonable compromise. Many doctors would disagree.

Sonia died three nights later, shortly after her family had gone home to get some rest. She underwent a short period of CPR, but it soon became clear that there was nothing imminently reversible, so the team quite rightly stopped.

The tone we should take with patients and their relatives has always vexed me. About seven years ago the playwright Alan Bennett wrote eloquently and amusingly about his experiences as an inpatient in UCH. Later, when he had fully recovered, he returned to the hospital to read some diary entries, thank the staff and take part in a question-and-answer session. He talked about his surprise when, during his pre-operative assessment interview, he was asked out of the blue whether he dyed his hair. 'No,' he'd replied. 'Why? Would it affect my chances if I did?'*

He also described the surreal experience of parading down to the operating theatre in a line with the other patients, all carrying their own pillows and notes, like monks on the way to chapel. He contrasted the sterile, lonely, single room of a private hospital with being surrounded by funny and inspiring fellow patients in an open bay in the NHS. He told us about the painful experience of listening to a 'very chatty and jokey' (and no doubt star-struck) consultant, when all he wanted was information, reassurance and to be left alone. We all smiled politely and nodded, but I was struck by the contradiction. He appreciated the company of his naturally funny 'salt-of-the-earth' fellow patients, but not the attempts at humour by his boorish doctor. It was a perfectly reasonable position – we all know people who make us feel tired as soon as they start speaking – but I felt sorry for the doctor. I am a big fan of Alan Bennett and I had decided to stay quiet and follow the old adage 'never meet your heroes', but now I couldn't help myself. My arm shot up.

'Do you think, then, that humour is best avoided?' I stammered. 'In a doctor.'

My inclination is to use humour. Often it seems to help, but perhaps I am kidding myself. He thought for a moment, smiled and then replied, 'It depends who you are, I suppose.'

Of course it does.

Some patients are just abusive (not Alan Bennett, obviously). Often it is because they are confused, mentally unwell or

* At the age of eighty-four Alan Bennett still had a shock of blond hair that the pre-assessment nurse, who'd never heard of him, couldn't quite believe. I am not aware that it has prognostic significance.

paranoid, but occasionally they are of completely sound mind and still vile to the staff. UCH has a strict zero-tolerance policy for such abuse, but often I find myself finessing it and making compromises.

A few years ago I walked up to a patient called Denise in Bed 20 on my Monday morning ward round to be greeted with, 'What do you fucking want, you fucking piece of shit? Don't come near me. I know what you're about.'

I tried to explain why I was there, but Denise was having none of it. She was an intravenous drug user in her mid-thirties and had been admitted the day before with a perforated duodenal ulcer. She'd sailed through the operation to repair the ulcer, but had come to the unit overnight for monitoring and had been persistently abusive to the staff.

'I'm not fucking staying,' she continued, sitting forward, 'not with you fucks. I'm fucking going. I want a smoke.'

The security guard who was permanently stationed by her bed twitched, but Denise slumped back into her sheets.

'I'm sorry, but you might die if you leave now,' I informed her from a safe distance. 'You've got tubes and lines sticking into you. Let me get the surgeons and then we'll try to get you outside for a cigarette.'

As I left the bay, I was approached by one of the senior nurses.

'We can't take her down for a cigarette. She's got a history of mental illness, she needs a psych nurse, it's the policy.'

My hackles rose. Denise was not mentally ill she was just angry, unpleasant and wanted a cigarette.

'And can you read her the zero-tolerance policy.'

'Sure,' I replied.

The zero-tolerance policy states that if a patient of sound mind is abusive and threatening we should deliver a verbal warning, then a written warning and finally, if they persist, exclude them from the hospital. I support it, but I didn't want to risk Denise's life by kicking her out of the hospital. I could just imagine the coroner's inquest . . .

'So tell me, why did Denise die?'

'Well, she was nasty to us and wouldn't listen to our warnings, so . . .'

Inevitably, Denise was as nice as pie to the surgeon, but when he left, her mood soured again and she demanded to go for that smoke, so we found a wheelchair and I offered to escort her (with the security guard). On our way down in the lift, I spotted a possible flaw in the plan.

'Have you got any cigarettes?' I asked.

'Don't worry about that,' she mumbled and, not relishing another verbal assault, I decided to take her advice.

It was a warm spring day and small groups of staff were chatting and enjoying the sun in the ambulance bay. I recognized a couple of nurses and nodded politely.

'Over there,' Denise growled, pointing at two men in their sixties who were smoking behind an ambulance. 'Take me there.'

I should have seen it coming, it was obvious, but for a moment I couldn't bring myself to drag Denise across the tarmac past my colleagues to help her beg for a cigarette. I felt like Lou to her Andy in the *Little Britain* sketch, but I was committed now, so after one more insistent growl, over we went.

Despite Denise's polite request, the two men hesitated. I sympathized; she looked as if one more fag might kill her. On the other hand, cigarettes would probably kill them too, eventually. They looked at me, so I shrugged, slightly pathetically, and out came their Rothmans.

Denise behaved much better after her cigarette. We even managed to discuss the zero-tolerance policy, although I think we both knew that I'd be unlikely to throw her out on the street. But I'd supported the nurses and kept Denise in hospital for another twenty-four hours at least. And I'd got ten minutes out in the sunshine.

Building relationships with patients and relatives is vital. Trust is a crucial part of that, so our starting position should be openness, but that does not mean about everything always. We mustn't be dishonest or patronizing, but neither should we cause unnecessary anguish and suffering. Patients will always be vulnerable, however much we empower them, because when our bodies fail us and we are faced with our own mortality it's frightening and we rely on others. I am not advocating paternalism, but good doctors judge how, when and, to an extent, what information to tell their patients, depending on the individual and the circumstances. We are not employed to be robots, we are expected to be empathetic and compassionate as well as honest and transparent.

I am often asked by relatives how their loved one died. I answer, 'peacefully', because it's true; we ensure that in modern ICU, but what if it was outside the hospital and the patient was scared, fighting for breath and in pain? Should I tell them that? Is there any point? Would you? If there is a reason to tell people things, or if they ask, then I do, but if there isn't and they don't ask I think about it much more carefully. We should give patients information for their benefit, not for ours or for any other reason – I think.

If patients really don't want to know the truth, then I think that's up to them – except it is not always that simple. Sometimes information has to be shared, whether the patient likes it or not, because future management depends upon it (in cases such as Carla's) or, as we shall see in the next chapter, because informed consent relies upon it.

11.   Capacity

Capacity and consent should be straightforward. To demonstrate capacity an adult has to pass four tests. They must understand the treatment options available, retain all the relevant information, weigh up the benefits and risks of the various alternatives and then communicate their decision back to the clinician. Informed consent requires that we explain the proposed treatment and the alternatives and then list all the material risks and benefits. An adult with capacity can then decide whether or not to consent to any treatments that we offer. Job done.

Following the case of *Montgomery* v. *Lanarkshire Health Board*,* the Bolam Test (that a reasonable body of medical peers would have acted in the same way – see Chapter 8) no longer applies to consent. Instead, doctors must provide information about 'all the "material risks" of an intervention, i.e. any risk to which a reasonable person in the patient's position would attach significance, or that this particular patient would be likely to attach significance.'

Capacity is decision specific. We don't necessarily have capacity to make all decisions or none; often we can make some but

---

* Mrs Montgomery was a small, diabetic woman who delivered a large baby vaginally. The baby suffered shoulder dystocia (got stuck) during delivery and suffered brain injury which led to cerebral palsy. Mrs Montgomery had raised concerns regarding vaginal delivery, but she had not inquired about the specific risks. Her obstetrician, Dr McLellan, believed that if she had been told of the specific risks (which were small) she would have opted for Caesarean section, but Dr McLellan believed that a vaginal delivery was the best option, so she did not mention the cerebral palsy risk. Mrs Montgomery won.

not others, depending on the complexity and consequences of the issues. One decision might be relatively simple to understand, but have very serious consequences, while another might be intellectually challenging but have only minor consequences. A patient can have capacity to make the first but not the second and vice versa.* The conclusion they come to, though, is irrelevant. As long as they pass the four tests they can decide to eschew conventional medicine and put their faith in herbs, hash and homeopathy if they want to. We can't go back and say, 'Well, they might have capacity officially, but they are clearly an idiot who doesn't know what's best for them, so let's pretend they didn't pass the tests.'

To deliver our treatment under those circumstances would be assault.

That all usually works well when patients are stable and in their right minds, but a person's capacity can vary over time with changes in their cognition and consciousness. This can become tricky when, having made one decision, a patient slips below the capacity threshold and changes their mind. At first glance it seems simple – no capacity no autonomy – but what about a woman in labour? Every anaesthetist in the country has come across a woman pleading for an epidural at three in the morning despite a birth plan in which she has clearly stated that she wants a natural birth and definitely no epidural (approximately half of people change their mind about pain relief during labour). She had capacity when she signed the plan before she went into labour, but now she is in pain, high on laughing gas and pethidine and sleep deprived. Can she really take on board the information, retain it, weigh up the risks and benefits and

---

* The Mental Capacity Act 2005 actually states that the capacity to make a decision relates only to the complexity of the decision, but in practice the gravity of the consequences affects how closely that capacity is examined.

then communicate that back to us? Does saying, 'Just put it in and stop patronizing me! I'm dying,' suffice?*

There is also asymmetry in the whole consent process because, while patients can refuse or accept treatments, they cannot demand them. Doctors are not compelled to deliver treatments that they deem futile. That seems reasonable, but it does uncover a subtle power imbalance and also points to other nuances and wrinkles in the process: the doctor is not impartial while the patient (and, indeed, usually the doctor) has not previously experienced any of the positive or negative outcomes of the planned intervention, so can only imagine what they are like, and humans are not logical.

Doctors offer treatments that they believe have a reasonable chance of benefit. For surgeons that is surgery, for gastroenterologists it's endoscopy and for oncologists it's chemotherapy, radiotherapy and immunotherapy. I don't think doctors deliberately influence patients towards a particular strategy, but they do influence them nevertheless. Doctors have all known patients that they desperately want to treat and others that they would prefer not to. The reason might be an emotional desire to help a desperate individual, fondness for a patient they've known for a long period, or a desire not to be saddled with either the blame for a bad outcome or the long-term care of a demanding and difficult one.† We fight hard to overcome these biases and they

* In practice we invariably override the birth plan and justify it in several ways. Firstly, an advance directive is only valid while the circumstances to which it pertains exist, so when a woman is in more pain than she'd envisaged, it could be considered void. Secondly, we are meant to act in a patient's best interests, and withholding effective pain control is not in the patient's best interests, and, finally, even if not capable of formal consent, the assent of a labouring woman could be considered a reasonable substitute.
† League tables will only exacerbate this. If our personal figures are in the public domain, then we will be even less willing to take on more tricky cases,

are not always harmful because our instincts are often correct, but it's important that we are aware of our own emotions and how they creep into the consent process.

'There are always risks, but I really think this will help you . . .'

'We could operate, but if I were you I'd avoid it for as long as you can . . .'

'In my experience facelifts are usually life changing.'

'I think you might be better being treated by someone closer to where you live . . .'

We can even influence people by the way we quote statistics. A 90 per cent chance of sailing through without a hitch is viewed much more positively than a 1 in 10 risk of a significant complication, and as soon as we mention death all bets are off. I might think that I relay the facts dispassionately, but I can tell by my emotional response to a patient's eventual choice that I do not. I am usually pleased or disappointed at the end of the conversation, which implies that I am almost certainly trying to persuade them one way or the other, even if only subconsciously.

And those realizations got me thinking more about the way patients make their decisions.

My dad has a consent form from the 1940s that says:

I consent to an operation.
Signed . . . .

That's it.

It prevented surgeons operating on people entirely against their will, I suppose, and I am attracted to its simplicity and honesty, but it does leave things a little open to interpretation.

Consent is now a process rather than a single event (I refuse to

---

because the ones that do badly will adversely affect our figures. The temptation to practise defensive medicine, i.e. medicine that protects us from criticism rather than delivers the best care to the patients, will be greater.

call it a journey), sought by a clinician who has detailed knowledge of the procedure and who explains the risks, benefits and alternatives. But the problem remains that, when faced with statistics, particularly about our own health, we are not good at making rational choices. Sometimes we struggle to make sense of the figures, sometimes we ignore the data and make emotional decisions, sometimes we are subliminally influenced by our clinician or family and sometimes there is no rational conclusion.

How do you weigh up the high chance of a small gain against the small chance of disaster? When do the benefits of replacing an arthritic knee joint outweigh the risks of the anaesthetic and surgery? When does the burden of weeks spent on intensive care outweigh the small chance of a longer life? Should we distinguish physical from psychological benefits? How many options should patients have? Is cosmetic surgery a special case? Can anyone meaningfully distinguish a risk of 1 in 1,000 from 1 in 10,000?

Perhaps this isn't the clinician's problem. Once we have presented the information our job is done. The patient's autonomy is paramount and people grapple with impossible decisions in all aspects of their life every day. In many ways this is no different. But this is a uniquely stressful moment for patients, and their doctors have a duty of 'care', not just a duty of 'inform and treat'. In the past we didn't give patients enough information and they probably trusted us too much, but perhaps today we have swung too far the other way. Patients want to trust us and they want us to communicate well, but that does not always equate to swamping them with huge amounts of information.

Any general anaesthetic can result in death. That must come under the umbrella of 'material risk', so when a young child comes into my anaesthetic room to be put to sleep for an appendectomy should I tell the parents that their child might die?

I think this would terrify most people and make some walk straight back out of the hospital. Of course, appendicitis is far more likely to kill their child, so I could balance the relative risks of death, but I don't think that would make them feel better. We don't expect the driver to tell us that we might die every time we get on a bus.

A few years ago I got a phone call from a non-medical university friend. He'd studied philosophy and had not got up before midday for three years (which still annoys me), but despite that, we'd kept in touch and now his wife was nine months pregnant. The conversation went something like this.

'Hey, Merl.' (He's called Merlin – don't ask me.) 'Any sign of a baby?'

'Yeah, boy, couple of hours ago.'

'Wonderful! Congratulations. Amazing! How's Katy?'

'She's . . . actually, that's why I'm calling.'

'Go on.' I was at work and had a patient waiting, but Merlin sounded anxious. He's usually horizontally relaxed.

'She needs to go to theatre because she's started bleeding, but the bloody anaesthetist's scared the life out of her.'

My hackles rose.

'I'm sure they . . . sorry, tell me.'

'He said something along the lines that because she's just had two helpings of shepherd's pie a general anaesthetic might well kill her, but her platelets are low so a spinal anaesthetic is likely to paralyse her. But if they do nothing she'll bleed to death, so . . .'

'Oh God. I'm sorry.'

This isn't going to sound great, but I sympathized with the anaesthetist. I could imagine him going through his options and seeing problems wherever he turned. During a general anaesthetic the large volume of shepherd's pie she'd just consumed might regurgitate into Katy's lungs and that *could* kill her; with a low platelet count she wouldn't form blood clots normally so she *could* bleed from the needle of a spinal anaesthetic, and that blood *could* compress the nerves below her spinal cord and cause paralysis; and letting Katy go on bleeding as she currently was, was obviously not an option. One might argue that the anaesthetist was just presenting the facts – doing his job.

'He looked terrified,' Merlin added. 'He was very young.'

'Yeah, look, don't worry, it'll be fine. He's just verbalizing his thought processes.'

'Great!'

'Ask if you can speak to the consultant anaesthetist on call. They'll sort it out – I promise.'

I don't know what the young anaesthetist actually said to my friends, but all they heard was 'paralysis or death'. He may have been gentle and tactful and he was in a difficult situation. He was duty bound to explain the risks and gain 'informed consent', but perhaps he allowed some of his own anxiety to permeate the conversation. I know that I have done that when I've been scared. In the end the consultant came in, smoothed the waters, slipped in a spinal anaesthetic and it was all fine. Katy can still walk and my godson is now a twenty-two-year-old body-building DJ with some impressive body art.

The chance of dying from an anaesthetic is about 1 in 80,000 across the population, and much lower if you are young and fit. So should we mention death to those anxious parents? However we phrase it, death is still death, and it's not a word that sits easily in a conversation about someone's child. The temptation is to use euphemisms – 'obviously everything in life carries risks' – followed by a knowing look and then, 'but anaesthetics are very safe these days'. Is that acceptable, or must I use the 'D' word?

A recent survey revealed that the worst thing about having an anaesthetic and operation for most people is the anxiety, worse than the pain or nausea or rehabilitation. Recounting in graphic detail the terrible things that might, extremely rarely, happen will protect the doctor in the single case in 80,000 when disaster strikes, but it will also add to the anxiety of the other 79,999. Is that a reasonable trade-off?

And what about when that child gets a bit older and starts to have opinions of their own? Then consent and capacity become even more complicated.

Up to the age of fifteen a child can only give consent to undergo a treatment if they are deemed to have adequate intelligence, competence and understanding of the risks and benefits (a criterion known as Gillick competence). Otherwise a responsible adult must give consent, although if a parent refuses, a court can overrule their decision in the best interests of the child. Sixteen- and seventeen-year-olds are assumed to have capacity, so they can give consent in the same way as an adult, but if they refuse a treatment and that refusal might lead to death or permanent injury their decision can be overruled by the Court of Protection. That still seems relatively clear and easy to follow, but when all the complexities collide the realities of consent and capacity can be confusing, fraught with dilemmas and occasionally troubling – as two teenagers with leukaemia that I looked after demonstrated.

Lauren was a gregarious, intelligent seventeen-year-old Jehovah's Witness. She was ambitious and had secured a place to study History at Oxford University (provided she got the A-level grades), but in 2019, just eight months before the exams, she was diagnosed with acute leukaemia. A month later she was on ICU. She'd responded well to the initial chemotherapy and her prognosis from the cancer was good, but the combination of the two had left her dangerously anaemic and she was adamant that she would not receive a blood transfusion. She was devout in her beliefs and, in line with Jehovah's Witness teaching, was convinced that accepting blood was against God's will and would lead to eternal damnation. That, in her opinion, was a fate worse than death so, even if her decision resulted in her demise, she planned to stick to it and she signed paperwork to that effect. The normal level of haemoglobin in the blood is between 120 and 160g/L. Lauren's was 38.

Haemoglobin, the molecule in red blood cells that carries oxygen, is usually 99 per cent saturated with oxygen in arteries, but only 75 per cent in veins, because by then 25 per cent has been offloaded to the tissues. Containing only 38g/L of haemo-globin, Lauren's blood could deliver less than a third as much oxygen as normal to her tissues, even if all those 38 grams were fully saturated. That put Lauren's vital organs at risk, and it was her heart that was first to show the strain. Already compromised by the chemotherapy and fluctuating salt levels, her heart could not handle the reduced oxygen supply and was flicking in and out of abnormal rhythms. It was also pumping less strongly than it should have been and, as well as looking white as a sheet, Lauren felt faint and was out of breath when she moved around her bed. Her low blood count was now contributing to a poten-tially life-threatening situation, and in normal circumstances we would have transfused blood at the same time as giving supple-mental oxygen and drugs to stabilize her heart.

We transferred Lauren down to the ICU for monitoring, gave her heart-stabilizing medication and used the opportunity to dis-cuss transfusion again. Perhaps faced with this complication she'd reconsider, we postulated, but her position didn't change. She did not want to receive blood, whatever the consequences. Her father had died when she was five, but her mother, also a devout Jeho-vah's Witness, supported her decision. She made it clear, however, that this was *Lauren*'s choice. She was terrified of losing her only daughter, but would support Lauren whatever she decided. Lau-ren's twenty-two-year-old brother, who had rejected the faith, was also often at the bedside, but it was clear that he wasn't going to try to change her mind. This was a discussion they'd already had – plenty of times – and he too respected her autonomy.

I wasn't directly looking after Lauren, I was on for the other side of the unit, but I remember feeling deeply frustrated by the thought of her dying at such a young age, unnecessarily. She was so bright and engaging and had so much to give, but my reaction was irrelevant; the only question was, did Lauren have the competence and capacity to refuse a blood transfusion?

Lauren passed all the standard tests of capacity (she understood the information, could retain it, weigh it and communicate her decision back to us), but she was only seventeen years old and her refusal to have blood might lead to her death, so we consulted the Trust's lawyers. They suggested that we request second opinions and a psychiatric assessment to ensure that Lauren had capacity and was not being coerced. Everyone agreed that she understood the consequences of the decision and she was not, so far as anyone could tell, being coerced by her mother or anybody else. We went back to the lawyers with this information and they advised that we honour Lauren's decision. If we and the psychiatrists were convinced that she had capacity and her mother was in agreement, then there was increasing case law to suggest that we should respect her wishes. She should not receive a blood transfusion, whatever the consequences.

We gave Lauren erythropoietin (EPO) to stimulate production of red blood cells, iron supplements, oxygen and fluids, and after three precarious days during which she lay listless and breathless as her monitor incessantly alarmed, she started to improve. Her heart rhythm settled, her blood count began to creep back up and each day she was able to do a little more. She did not receive a blood transfusion. Ten days later we discharged her from ICU to the general ward and there she continued to make a good recovery. She was always gracious and polite, and by the time she left the unit her sharp wit and bubbly personality had returned. Alongside a huge sense of relief, there was a general feeling among the staff that we had done the right thing, but I felt unsure. What if Lauren had died? We had all thought that that was possible – probable, even, at one point – but she didn't, so she walked away leaving her death as merely hypothetical.

It had been a stressful experience, so we scheduled a meeting to talk it through afterwards and to see whether there was anything we could learn. The meeting overran because people expressed a range of ethical opinions, experiences and arguments, but, crucially, everyone was relaxed. There was no stress because nothing bad had happened. She'd survived. There was no grieving parent, no angry older brother, no tortured nurses and no one interested in criticizing us. Despite following procedure throughout, we felt as though we'd been lucky and, as always, the outcome had affected our interpretation of events. So we just left it. We didn't go back to the lawyers and scrutinize their advice and we didn't change any processes or policies, we just had a civilized, hypothetical, ethical debate and then went about our business. But I couldn't get out of my head the fact that everything would have been different if Lauren had died. When I looked at it through that lens I was worried.

Why? Did I want to go against her wishes and give her blood? I wasn't sure. Competent adults have autonomy and as part of that they are allowed to make unwise choices, but was Lauren a competent adult? She was highly intelligent so there was no question that she could deal with the intellectual complexity of the decision, but that did not mean that she had the maturity and independence of thought to make a decision with such profound possible consequences. This could have meant death for Lauren, and that might have had lifelong consequences for many people around her.

I support the right to believe whatever you want, as long as it does not harm others, and I have no quarrel with Jehovah's Witnesses as a group. They have always been collaborative and sympathetic as we have jointly navigated areas of medicine that encroach upon their beliefs and they sponsor excellent medical research. I am uncomfortable, however, when any doctrine affects the treatment of children. A paediatric intensive-care colleague told me that they do not describe their patients as Christian children or Muslim children or, indeed, children of any religion. The parents may belong to a religious group but, until the children are old enough to decide for themselves, the treatments delivered are not influenced by creed. The staff are sensitive to cultural and religious customs and beliefs, but when it comes to life-altering medical interventions, they believe that their duty is to do what is in that child's best interests, whatever the family's background. This becomes more complex when a child's acceptance within a community is threatened by a medical intervention, because the psychological and social impact must be considered, but I believe it's a good starting principle.

The difficulty with Lauren was that I didn't know how limited her life experiences were and I didn't know how limited was too limited. Most of her life had been spent in a household of devout Jehovah's Witnesses, so had she had sufficient opportunity to consider alternative beliefs? I appreciate that we are all more likely to stay with the religion of our parents than to shop around for another, so there is an argument that few of us ever make fully independent, objective decisions. All our choices are influenced by our own anecdotal experiences and emotions, and 'availability bias' (the preponderance to be influenced by something we can easily bring to mind), is powerful. We are far less rational than we like to believe, which is why we make so many bad decisions, but I don't argue with our right to make them. The alternative is worse, so had Lauren been eighteen I would not have questioned her decision. I might have felt sad and frustrated, but I'd have accepted it. The reasons behind it would have been none of my business.

But she wasn't eighteen, she was seventeen, and although the distinction might seem arbitrary, in law there is a clear distinction.

Equally, had she been eight years old the situation would have been clear-cut. I would have sought permission from the Court of Protection to give the blood, even against her mother's wishes. She would have been too young to refuse potentially life-saving treatment and, if granted permission, I would have delivered the transfusion in her best interests.

So when do we become competent in these circumstances? When do our religious beliefs stop being our parents' and become our own? Is it on our eighteenth birthday? Or sixteenth? Or is it when we can convince a psychiatrist or a lawyer that we know our own minds? There was no evidence that Lauren's mother was anything other than loving towards her, but presumably at some point Lauren had been taught that having a blood transfusion would lead to eternal damnation. It could be argued that by not contradicting this her mother had effectively dissuaded her from agreeing to the transfusion, and so was putting her life at risk. We all expose our children to risk every day by taking them on car journeys and allowing them on trampolines, so the level of risk and the risk-to-benefit ratio is crucial, but standing by while a child refuses a potentially life-saving medical treatment worries me. Her older brother had received the same upbringing, but had rejected the religion at the age of eighteen. It was possible, although it didn't seem likely, that Lauren would do the same.

The philosophical arguments around this case are endless and unsolvable. There will always be different opinions about what choices teenagers should and shouldn't be allowed to make. The law has tried to find a way through it with the Mental Capacity Act and the Children Act, but grey areas remain. Lauren was a seventeen-year-old who had been brought up within a belief system that suggested she should sacrifice her life rather than accept a blood transfusion and now her life was in danger. For that reason I felt that legal advice was not enough. In my opinion, the highest authority possible, a judge from the Court of Protection, should have decided whether she had capacity. Had they concluded that she didn't, then we would have had to forcibly restrain an intelligent, lucid seventeen-year-old and deliver a treatment against her will. (There would also, of course, have been a complete loss of trust between the patient and her clinicians, which would have made ongoing treatment difficult, to say the least.) I have never done that and I hope that I never have to, but, equally, I've never sat by and watched a seventeen-year-old die of a treatable complication.

I suspect that a judge in the Court of Protection would have come to the same conclusion as the Trust's lawyers, and I would have gone along with their decision, whatever it was. But I'm still not sure what I'd have done if it had been purely up to me.

The other patient was Samuel, in many ways a typical fifteen-year-old. He was bright, a talented golfer, and had strong opinions, but four years previously he too had been diagnosed with leukaemia. He'd undergone chemotherapy and a bone-marrow transplant, but unfortunately had suffered a relapse and so in 2021 he came back into UCH to prepare for his final throw of the dice, chimeric antigen receptor or CAR T cells. CAR T-cell therapy is a novel treatment that involves taking the patient's own T cells (a type of white blood cell that fights infection), altering them so that they will attack a receptor on the cancer cells, multiplying up the number of cells in the lab and then returning them. Essentially, it is a method of reprogramming and turbocharging the patient's own immune system to kill off the cancer. At the time of writing it is an established treatment for a limited number of blood cancers and being trialled in several others. But it can have serious side effects, so CAR T patients need close monitoring, sometimes in ICU. It was Samuel's last chance of a cure and, if undertaken in optimal conditions, offered him a 30 to 40 per cent chance of survival. He knew the odds and spoke frankly (as was his style) to his parents on their way down from their home in Northampton about the possibility of not surviving.

Samuel was up on the adolescent ward, halfway through preparatory disease-reducing treatment, when, in the early hours of a Saturday morning in April, he had a seizure. The haematology doctors controlled it with diazepam (Valium) and then loaded him with levetiracetam (Keppra), an antiseizure medication, but within an hour he'd had two more.

Seizures are caused by abnormal electrical activity in the brain. This can be the result of many things: imbalance of the salts, low sugar levels, infection, bleeding, high temperature, tumours, repeated flashing lights or sleep deprivation. Anything that changes the milieu of the brain cells can result in abnormal electrical firing and a seizure. The external manifestations of that seizure depend on where the abnormal activity occurs. If it is generalized then we lose consciousness and have a classic 'tonic-clonic' (shaking and stiffness) seizure, but if it occurs in just one area of the brain the signs may be localized to whatever activity that particular part controls. Samuel's seizure was generalized.

Having checked his salts, sugar and oxygen levels and added another antiseizure drug, Samuel's haematology team sent him down for a CT scan. He had a low platelet count, so there was a risk that he'd bled into his brain, and the CT confirmed several small patches of fresh blood scattered through the brain tissue. These were causing localized swelling, but otherwise the brain looked structurally normal. So far, no permanent damage had been done. He was still drowsy after the scan, so we gave him extra platelets and admitted him to ICU for monitoring. Either the seizures themselves or the diazepam used to terminate them explained the initial drowsiness, but as the morning progressed, rather than waking up, he became more sleepy. By mid-afternoon he was making noises rather than speaking and only opening his eyes in response to a painful stimulus. Every so often his face contorted into a grimace and he lifted his hands to either side of his head, so we repeated the CT scan and discovered, as feared, that despite the platelets he had continued to bleed. Now his whole brain was being squashed by the blood and he was in serious danger. Further bleeding would put pressure on the base of Samuel's brain, and when that happened there would be no way back. It was a desperate situation.

We transfused more bags of platelets and telephoned the paediatric neurosurgeons at Great Ormond Street hospital. The only way to reduce the pressure on his brain now was to remove an area of skull and allow it to expand. The neurosurgeons said they'd be willing to try this, so while the team prepared to put him to sleep, take over his breathing and set up the transfer, I sat down with the on-call consultant haematologist and, via telephone, Samuel's primary consultant to discuss whether what we were proposing was the right thing to do.

Several factors were in play. Sustaining this much brain injury and then undergoing surgery would put his leukaemia treatment schedule under threat. He still needed more disease-reducing therapy prior to the CAR T cells, but that would now need to be delayed by a week at least, probably longer. He'd then have to make an almost miraculous recovery, which would take a month at the very least, to be strong enough for CAR T, and all that time the leukaemia would be progressing. Added to that, his brain injury was life changing. However well the surgery went, he'd never fully recover to be the person he was before, and in someone with all Samuel's problems, the surgery itself was fraught with danger. But he was fifteen years old. He had a potentially long life ahead of him and without the surgery he would certainly die, so we came to the conclusion that, if the neurosurgeons were prepared to operate, then we should pass that on to Samuel's parents as an option. He would be asleep, so he wouldn't suffer, and we could review our decision if the circumstances changed.

'What if the parents say no?' I asked.

'Then we respect their wishes,' his primary consultant replied without hesitation. 'It's a completely reasonable choice.'

As we walked down the corridor to meet Samuel's parents I asked the consultant haematologist how she thought they would react to the news.

'They'll be calm,' she said. 'Upset, obviously, but they will listen, talk it through and come to a joint decision. At least, they always have done up to now.'

'Right.'

I was doubtful. They might have been calm before, but this was different, surely.

But I was wrong. Samuel's mother and father behaved exactly as my colleague had predicted. After we had explained the findings of the CT scan and the offer of surgery, they asked a couple of questions and then began an extraordinary dialogue.

For the next twenty minutes, my colleague and I listened to one of the most compassionate and brave discussions we'd ever heard. They began by confirming to each other that they both understood what had happened and then questioned whether surgery was the right option. They talked about the four years of treatment that Samuel had been through and about how hard it had been for him both physically and emotionally. Their faces glowed with love and pride, as they described his bravery and defiance, the sporting tournaments he had won and the joy he had brought them. But they were also candid. Samuel had known that he was in desperate trouble when the leukaemia had returned after the bone-marrow transplant and he'd made it clear that he would not relish a life with severe disability. He was a force of nature, a light that burned bright, a feisty teenager who'd grabbed life and dealt with everything it had thrown at him, but he wasn't interested in just existing. His parents were in no doubt that if he couldn't be *him* then he'd rather not be. He'd go through whatever it took, but only if the prize at the end was worth suffering for.

Time and again Samuel's parents dismissed their own feelings to concentrate on what was best for their son – what he would choose. I know this because they verbalized everything. There was no filter, everything they thought, they said. Perhaps most impressively, they projected into the future. They were aware of the magnitude of the decision and they knew that they would return to this moment for years to come, whichever choice they made, with regrets and doubts.*

Gradually it became clear that Samuel's parents were going to decline surgery, but they didn't rush the decision. As one of them seemed to make up their mind, they'd spot a glimmer of doubt in the other and so pause to allow their partner time to express or process their concerns. They addressed every aspect

---

* The psychologist Gary Klein's term 'pre-mortem' describes a process for businesses who are faced with a big decision. He suggests they hire experts to project a year into the future before they proceed. In the projected future the choice they have made is a disaster. The idea of the exercise is to examine what that disaster looks like before they finally commit to a course of action. Samuel's parents were going through a similar process.

of the situation with clarity and compassion. They spoke openly about the impact of the previous four years on Samuel and on them and their other children. They considered all the possible outcomes and for a while they clung again to the tiny possibility of recovery. But then they weighed it against the terrible odds and the huge burden of future treatments and reflected on all the pain and anguish that he had suffered and on all his hopes, dreams and disappointments.

In the end they returned to a simple question.

'A part of me just wants to fight for him and try anything,' his mother said, 'however grim it looks, but . . . is that right for him? Is that what he would want?'

As she spoke, I tried to put myself in their shoes. Our twins were eleven at the time, just turning into complicated, unique individuals showing glimpses of what they might become in the future. What would I do? It was impossible to know, of course, because I had not been through all they and Samuel had over the previous four years, but I thought that I'd have gone for surgery. Even if I knew that the chance of success was negligible, while heroics were being offered, I couldn't imagine opting for palliation. I would have been clinging to anything to postpone the horror of losing a child – I think.

Eventually they settled on the decision to concentrate on Samuel's comfort and dignity and allow nature to take its course. They sat quietly for a moment, letting the choice settle, and then looked at each other and nodded. They were convinced that this is what he would have chosen.

As I walked away from the relatives' room, I began to question myself. Should we have allowed them to make this decision on behalf of their child? If we thought that there was even a tiny chance of some degree of recovery, should we have insisted on surgery? I felt that increasingly familiar knot of anxiety. What if we'd got this wrong? When I spoke to the neurosurgeons they were surprised by the parents' decision, which added to my unease, but when I relayed the family discussion to Samuel's primary consultant, she described their choice as courageous. She knew, deep down, that Samuel had reached the end of the line, but she'd been clinging to any glimmer of hope. It's usually the clinicians who persuade the families about the reality of these desperate situations, but in this case it took those closest to Samuel, his family, who loved him more than anything in the world, to show us.

Samuel died the next day, peacefully in his sleep, with his family at the bedside holding his hands and reminding him how much they loved him.

Remembering these two cases stirs up a complicated mixture of emotions. I feel desperately sad for Samuel's family, but also inspired by them and at peace with the decision we all made. I believe wholeheartedly that we did what Samuel would have wanted and what was in his best interests. It was heartbreaking and stressful at the time, but I have no regrets. In Lauren's case, however, although with the benefit of hindsight we did the right thing by her, the successful outcome owed as much to luck as to judgement. She both survived and avoided blood, so the result was perfect, and I am delighted about that, but we didn't know that she'd survive when we decided to respect her wishes. That still bothers me.

These examples might seem extreme, but they highlight how complex and delicate issues around capacity and consent can be. The GMC and the courts are right to prioritize patient autonomy in the consent process, but ICU patients often lack capacity, so decisions have to be made in their best interests by other people. Many argue that we should all be encouraged to write advanced directives when we are well to cover what we would and wouldn't want in different circumstances. I agree that it should be an option, but I would hesitate to write my own.* The difficulty is making decisions about our future selves. What constitutes an acceptable quality of life for a twenty-year-old has often changed by the time they are seventy, and I don't know what I will want if I am stuck on a ventilator in multiple organ failure in twenty years' time. At the moment I've got a lot to live for, and my default position is that I would want everything to be done, but if I suffer a stroke next week and end up on the unit with significant brain injury, I want the doctors and my family to wrestle with what they think is best for me. That might sound selfish, but it's honest. I don't believe in the sanctity of life regardless of circumstances, but neither do I feel capable of saying what would and wouldn't be an acceptable quality of life for me in different situations and at different points in the future.

My mother's dementia progressed rapidly through 2021, and towards the end of the year the manager of her nursing home asked my father whether he thought she should be for CPR. Mum had always hinted that she'd not want to be wired up to machines, although she'd never made a formal advanced directive and obviously she couldn't now. But our whole family agreed that she should not be for CPR and a form was signed. A couple of months later she deteriorated again and ended up bed-bound. She'd stopped eating, was losing weight rapidly and was sleeping most of the time, so now the team asked whether we thought she should be for hospital treatment if she developed

---

* For patients in hospital or in the community with severe or terminal diseases we write Treatment Escalation Plans (e.g. 'for antibiotics and fluids but not for ventilation', or, 'for full escalation of organ support') in collaboration with them or their family to ensure that the on-call team do not do the 'wrong thing' in the middle of the night. These are vital, but even they come unstuck when circumstances or treatments we'd not considered crop up or when patients change their minds.

an infection, or for comfort measures in the nursing home. It was devastating to see my wonderful, vibrant mother so reduced, but again we all agreed that she'd not have wanted to go to hospital in these circumstances. However, as I sat by her bed watching her slip away, I felt panicky. I had an overwhelming sensation that I was letting her down and wanted to scoop her up and take her to an ICU. I knew it was crazy, but suddenly in the moment I couldn't bear the thought of losing her. Tish talked me down and eventually I accepted that we just needed to be there. It was horrible, but we couldn't change the situation, I knew in my heart that we'd made the right decision and I didn't begrudge Mum not writing an advanced directive. She died peacefully the next day, and in the end it was a huge relief to see her suffering over.

So sorry, Tish, Tom and Edie, I am not going to write an advanced directive. On the plus side, it is a compliment – I trust you. Officially, in hospital, these treatment escalation decisions are the responsibility of the doctors, of course, but remember, Tish, that, if they want to turn me off, you can challenge them – in the courts if necessary.

When patients have capacity, clinicians strive to give them accurate information so that they can make informed decisions, but to contend that we do it objectively is naive. Doctors influence patients and their relatives, both consciously and subconsciously, because doctors are humans with emotions and opinions. It is unavoidable and some patients love it.

'Whatever you think, Doctor. I am in your hands' is still a phrase that most doctors hear every day.

There is no easy fix, but awareness is the first step. The more cognizant we are of our own biases and assumptions, the more rigorous we are in assessing capacity, and the more we strive to be objective, the better the process will be.

But I hope that there will always be a place to request medical 'advice'. We don't buy medical care off the internet, we take ourselves to professionals, listen to their expertise and (usually) follow their advice. We talk a lot about 'patient-centred care', which seems a given (who else would the care be centred on?), but treatment plans emerge from a delicate and complex interaction. The duty of the doctor is to be diligent, compassionate and equitable, and to respect the wishes of the patient. The vast majority of doctors strive to achieve this every day, but it involves judgement and intuition. We are getting better at it, but let's not pretend that controversies around capacity and consent are confined to the past. And let's not be afraid to seek out the expertise of judges and others when things get really difficult.

12. Pandemic

On some days I can almost forget that it ever happened. The old rhythms of the unit have returned. The bed pressures, the worrying cases, the frustrating frequent-flyer patients and the complex family dynamics are all back and the stress levels ebb and flow as they always have. If it weren't for the staff absences, the incidental positive tests and the security guards on the front door handing out masks, I could kid myself that we are back to normal. But dig a little deeper and it's clear that Covid has changed ICU, and the people who work there, for ever.

There have undoubtedly been positives. The light shone on intensive care led to a welcome expansion in our bed base and it increased the number of applicants to medical and nursing school and to training in ICU specifically, but the pandemic had a mixed impact on the incumbent ICU staff. Some relished the challenge and flourished and some seemed to carry on unperturbed, but many were worn down by it over the months and eventually left their jobs in search of less harrowing work. For me, personally, it was a rollercoaster, like a whole career concertinaed into a few months.

The build-up was all about fear and anticipation. How many patients would come in and how much risk would I be at personally? A huge sense of shared purpose was matched by my individual, largely unspoken, apprehension. As we prepared, practised and planned for every eventuality, redeployed staff, redistributed equipment and built new ICUs, my anxiety grew. But when it finally hit, the reality of Covid took me by surprise. Worries about my own health quickly dissipated as I learnt to trust the PPE, and although the numbers were huge (despite being mitigated by the lockdowns), it was the illness itself that shocked me most. It was a brand-new virus, so, obviously, we didn't know what to expect, but I'd thought it would be roughly comparable to other ICU lung infections. I didn't expect to be facing the most severe, protracted, unpredictable pathogen I'd ever encountered. It was one thing to triple the size of our unit, but quite another to then fill it with this disease.

Clinically, we did all the things we usually do. We put in lines, used tight CPAP masks, sedated and ventilated when we needed to, took over the work of the kidneys and supported the blood pressure, but the patients with Covid didn't respond to these interventions in the usual way. Their low oxygen levels didn't fit with their clinical symptoms, some of them became terrifyingly inflamed for no discernible reason and they formed far more blood clots than they should have. Many continued to deteriorate inexorably despite everything we did, while others clung on to life for weeks when by normal criteria they should have succumbed. We were forced to question things we thought we knew and adjust our clinical strategies on the hoof. And as we did so we were acutely aware that every ICU in the world was treating this one disease – each of them slightly differently. What if our approach was wrong?

I found it unnerving and exhausting, not least because there were so many aspects to consider. Should we keep it simple and safe or try to be clever? Should we offer the highest level of care to a small number or more basic care to many? Would we run out of ventilators first or oxygen – or staff? But even standard clinical issues we'd dealt with throughout our careers became warped and confused by this baffling new virus: fundamental things, such as judging when to put someone on a ventilator, when to thin their blood and when artificial support had become futile and it was time to stop. Covid patients just did not follow the rules.

Initially, arguments raged about all these issues, but soon the ICU community began to collaborate on an unprecedented scale. Research groups joined forces to run trials of multiple different interventions and picked out those that were most effective within months. National bodies such as the Intensive Care Society issued guidance at record speed, newly established expert transfer teams moved critically sick Covid patients between hospitals and the ICUs formed networks and communicated with each other several times a day to discuss who needed to be moved where.

Covid put us on the map and changed our relationship with the public. Having previously been a scary black box that most people didn't really want to look inside, for a period ICU became the number-one topic of conversation. The world was worrying about ventilators, the UK government was building 4,000-bedded ICUs in exhibition centres and many people were terrified that they'd end up in one of those beds. Suddenly everyone knew what ICU was, but their opinion of us and Covid changed over time.

We began the pandemic as heroes. When most of the country were asked to retreat into their homes to protect themselves and others, we were tasked to do the opposite. And every Thursday we were given a round of applause for it. The clapping was for supermarket workers and bus drivers as well, of course (who turned out to be putting themselves at far higher risk than ICU staff), but in the hierarchy of heroic jobs, ICU doctor was beaten only by ICU nurse. We were the soldiers on the front line, the guardians of the people. We were putting our own lives in danger to save the country from this invisible adversary. It was our fifteen minutes of fame. Even Andy Murray talked about medicine as an alternative career. And the hospital was a scaled-down version of society at large. Intensive care was top of the tree. Everyone was reporting to the intensivists to ask what they could do to help. It was a strange, unsettling experience.

Of course, our celebrity didn't last. When it became clear that Covid would not be over in three months, but instead might go on indefinitely, our star began to fall. People got fed up with lockdowns and wanted to get on with their lives. The financial hardships kicked in, parents tired of home schooling, GCSEs and A levels were in chaos, there was a secondary mental-health crisis and ICU was no longer the priority. Most people were still sympathetic and grateful, but the country was ready to move on – and it was no different in the hospital. There was a huge backlog of operations and outpatient appointments and the extra hassle and complexity of separating Covid from non-Covid and possible-Covid made everyone irritable. They all just wanted their old lives back.

Many of the public were still cautious, but many weren't, and a whole new breed of 'experts' emerged. Suddenly half the country were epidemiologists, immunologists, virologists and pharmacologists. Journalists proclaimed without an ounce of doubt that lockdowns were a waste of time, that masks didn't work, that the mental-health crisis would kill far more people than Covid itself, that antiparasite drugs or antimalarials were miracle Covid cures, or that the pandemic was having no impact on life expectancy because it was only killing people after they should already have died (by dint of the fact that the average age of death from Covid was above the national life expectancy). Some of these claims were obviously nonsense (those who died of Covid lost on average ten years of life), and others such as antimalarials and antiparasite agents have been rigorously investigated and disproved, while the remainder continue to be fiercely debated.

Sometimes, however, the strength of spurious opinion directly affected our ability to do our job.

By the end of the second big surge most of the Covid patients on ICU were those who'd decided not to get vaccinated, often following the advice of a family member. That same family member might then request that, rather than use the approved drugs (such as dexamethasone or tocilizumab), we treat their loved one with ivermectin (an antiparasite drug), hydroxychloroquine (an antimalarial) or another favourite drug of their group. Finally, they'd object to our plan to sedate and ventilate their relative when the time came, not because their family member wouldn't have wanted everything, but because they had been reliably informed that ventilating Covid patients killed them.

All of this was usually done politely and with the best of intentions, but it made our jobs much more complicated. All aspects of Covid, including the management in ICU, were now part of the national debate. As with every other element of the pandemic, people had become polarized, entrenched in their camps, secure in their echo chambers and suspicious of experts and professionals. They were the minority, but unfortunately a disproportionate number of them or their families ended up in ICU.

The scale of the tragedy caused by Covid shocked us at the time, of course, but in 2021, after the second big wave, I was given a new insight into just how cruel it had been.

Families could not visit during Covid, except at critical moments such as intubation or end of life, so initially we tried to update them on the telephone. That proved to be unreliable and impractical, so quickly we set up a new group, the Family Liaison Team (FLT). Their job was to act as a point of contact and support for families, to ensure that they were kept up to date with progress and to arrange virtual visits to the bedside using iPads. The FLT were brilliant, and in 2021 they linked with the Quality Improvement Group to conduct a survey of those families and find out what it had really been like. There follows a small sample of what the relatives had to say:

'He passed by himself. This eats away at me.'

'You know what really gets me? That whole time, all those wonderful people who looked after my mum, I never knew who they were. I never saw their faces. She spent her last few weeks on earth with people I wouldn't recognize walking down the street and I wasn't there.'

'You can't understand what it meant to see someone hold her hand or wipe the hair out of her eyes.'

'Our lives were dictated by phone calls: We would pray that the phone would ring, so we would have an update, hoping she would have improved. Then we would pray the phone wouldn't ring.'

'I want closure, not on my wife, but on her death. I need to be able to have all the information to be able to process it. I don't understand how she waved goodbye to me in the ambulance and weeks later she was dead.'

'We saw how happy the people were that were looking after him when he was getting better. They really seemed happy. They sent us photos the first time he stood up. It makes you cry.'

Every response was poignant and many were heartbreaking, but some also took me by surprise. Before then I had never paused to consider how important it was for the families to see our faces. I knew that phone updates were not ideal. More than half of communication is non-verbal, so expecting us to build the same relationships down the telephone was hopelessly naive, but for some reason I'd thought we just would. However, listening to the impact of handing over the care of your critically sick, sometimes dying loved one to people you wouldn't recognize in the street, really hit home. No wonder it was hard for them to develop trust.

I was and still am largely dismissive of the antimask campaign. It feels belligerent, reactionary and selfish, a minor inconvenience pitted against a serious public health hazard, but I think I underestimated the impact that masks can have on communication and emotional connection. Sometimes when people are at their most vulnerable they need to see our whole faces (not just our eyes), so that we become recognizable human beings for them to put their faith in. I know that some clinicians occasionally removed their masks to break down the barriers. At the time I thought they were foolhardy, but now I admire their bravery and selflessness, because I think the benefit to the relative or patient may have justified the risk. I don't think it justified the risk in shops, on trains, or even in most health-care settings, but very occasionally the emotional power of showing your face might have been worth it. I was never brave enough to do it myself.

The relatives also talked about the impact of the media coverage on their suffering. We'd allowed the BBC to film in our ICU because we believed that conveying the public health message – Stay at home! – was vital, but the images on TV were shocking for the families. The ICU looked terrifying and we told the reporters that we were stretched to breaking point and barely able to cope. To an extent, we wanted to shock people. We wanted them to realize how serious the situation was so that they'd follow the rules, but we didn't think about the impact on the families of patients already in ICU. Most had not been able to visit, so their first impression of a Covid ICU was the one we gave them on the six o'clock news. Wondering whether the care of your wife or husband was being affected by the pressure on the system must have been awful.

★

The true impact of Covid on ICU will become clear only over time. There will be positives; improved collaboration between units and research groups, expansion in the number of beds and better public understanding of ICU, to name a few, but there will be negatives as well, including the long-term effects on staff. The impact it had on me was complicated. It made me more confident about the importance of ICU and the positive impact that doing it well can have on patients and their families (whatever the outcome), but it also left me with more questions, guilt, doubt and insecurity than I'd ever faced before. The speed, scale and severity of the two big waves were (and still are) hard to comprehend, and as I stumbled out the other side I felt dazed. There was too much to compute; too much suffering, tragedy and uncertainty and too many unknowns, what ifs and if onlys. Like countless colleagues, I was haunted by many of the patients I'd met and some of the decisions I'd made. I wasn't sleeping well, I was jumpy and I was short-tempered around the kids, but life and work went on. They had to.

13. Crash

By April 2021 the second big wave of Covid had died down. The still expanded unit was running at roughly ten critically sick Covid patients at a time alongside, but carefully separated from, thirty non-Covid ICU patients. The virus continued to shock, confuse and appal us on a regular basis, but we were also trying to get back to normal, or 'new' normal, whatever that would prove to be. We were all gradually returning to the pre-pandemic elements of our job, but I'd barely delivered an anaesthetic for over a year so I was nervous about working in the operating theatre. It was great to be treating non-Covid patients, but my muscle memory had gone and I had to concentrate harder than usual, even on simple procedures. I noticed that I was checking everything more than usual: double checking that my anaesthetic machine was fully functional, reconfirming the patients' allergies one extra time and looking back through the ICU charts that I'd studied only hours before.

Linda was fifty-six. She had thin dark hair, scraped back into a scruffy pony tail, and pale puffy skin punctuated by liver spots and broken veins. She was an alcoholic, often discovered unconscious and occasionally combative in the local park, and was well known to the Emergency Department, but she had a loving brother and son and, when sober, was disarmingly witty and perceptive. I'd met her a year previously when she'd come to the unit for monitoring after a particularly heavy drinking session and I'd liked her. The next day there'd been no bed up on the ward so Linda had been stuck on ICU and, before taking herself off home (against medical advice), she'd spent the day observing and evaluating the staff dynamics. On the ICU ward round she pointed out to me all sorts of things I hadn't noticed in fifteen years of working there – the glance between the trainee doctors when I requested something that they didn't agree with, the power dynamics between the physios and the nurses, the subtle favours asked and returned and the silent and pretty much unregarded backbone of support offered by cleaners and caterers. She'd left me feeling enlightened and a bit paranoid.

Now she was back. It was nearly midnight on a Monday and Linda had arrived in the ED earlier that evening, mildly inebriated. She'd come in because of three days of abdominal pain and vomiting. Her blood pressure was low, her pulse-rate high and she was running a mild fever. A bedside arterial blood gas showed that her blood was acidic with a high lactate level, usually a sign that either an area of the body is not receiving enough oxygen or that the liver is failing.

The ICU registrar, Matt (efficient and unassuming with some impressively intricate tattoos), had reviewed her in the ED at 9 p.m. and then phoned me to discuss the plan. She looked 'sick', Matt confirmed, but the cause was not clear. She was pale and drowsy, with cold hands and feet and a tender abdomen. We agreed that she needed fluid resuscitation in the ED initially, along with pain relief, antibiotics (in case she'd developed sepsis), a central venous line through which to give drugs for the low blood pressure and an arterial line (in the wrist) to monitor that blood pressure beat to beat. After that he would bring her to the ICU via a CT scan of her chest, abdomen and pelvis. With a bit of luck, that would give us the diagnosis.

At 11.45 p.m. I turned off my bedside light. I'd tried to call Matt at 11.30, but it had gone straight to voicemail so I'd decided to get some sleep. My phone was on charge by the bed, I'd arranged my pillows into the usual L shape to support my elbow that no longer straightens and stretched out my lower back. Tish was playing solitaire on her phone, but the screen blurred as my eyes closed.

'Night, love,' I mumbled.

'Night.'

The phone made both of us jump. As expected, it was Matt, but he didn't have the news I'd been hoping for. Linda was now up on the unit in Bed 16, a dark, cramped corner of Bay 1, and Matt had carried out our plan to the letter. He'd given Linda four litres of intravenous fluid (a generous dose), but despite that, her blood pressure was still falling, her lactate level rising and she was making only dribbles of urine. Most worryingly, the CT scan did not offer an explanation. Our CT scans are reported remotely overnight by radiologists in Australia, which has a certain logic because it's their daytime, but it does make the whole process a bit impersonal. Linda's report stated that the blood supply to the bowel, liver, kidneys and other major organs looked fine and that there was no evidence of bowel blockage or perforation, or of pancreatitis. The liver was shrunken and irregular, so almost certainly cirrhotic from the alcohol, but that on its own was not the answer. In the chest there was a small amount of fluid between the left lung and the chest wall, but otherwise nothing dramatic. There was no evidence of pneumonia and no large blood clots in the arteries to her lungs (pulmonary emboli). One by one my potential diagnoses had gone by the wayside. There was no escaping it, I needed to go in.

As I drove to the hospital I tried to work out what on earth could be going on. Linda was in shock – a state of low blood pressure and inadequate circulation to the vital organs. Already her kidneys were shutting down, she was drowsy (implying that her brain was struggling) and her liver function was abnormal. I ran through the different causes of shock: there was no evidence of bleeding (her blood count was rock steady, despite all the fluid), there was no indication of spinal or neurological damage and she had none of the other signs of anaphylaxis. It had to be either infection or the heart.

By the time I got there Matt had managed to dig up some more recent information about Linda that I'd been unaware of. She had been on the ICU of a different hospital four months previously with an infected leg ulcer, sepsis and liver failure. For much of her four-week stay they had not thought she would recover, but she'd finally turned the corner with powerful antibiotics and ICU support. Her recovery on the ward had been slow, however, because her poor liver function meant that she'd been intermittently drowsy and confused, and she had only made it home six weeks ago. Could this all be sepsis again?

There was a funny atmosphere on the unit that night. As ever, the lights were dimmed and the nurses were moving around quietly and efficiently, but they seemed listless. When I greeted people I was met with a nod and a grunt rather than a smile and a quip about how it was surely past my bedtime. The junior doctors seemed hassled and irritable, and when I popped into the coffee room to check in with the nurse in charge, the people on their break weren't talking to each other. They were all sitting separately, engrossed in their phones.

I dumped my jacket behind the front desk, rolled up my sleeves, pulled on an FFP3 mask and pushed open the door to Bay 1. The other patients were quiet, two sedated on ventilators, one gently snoring on high-flow oxygen and the other, a forty-five-year-old man who'd had his large bowel removed that day because of a flare-up of his ulcerative colitis, plugged into something on his iPad. All the activity was around Linda. Her nurse, Daniel, was moving around the bed, drawing up drugs, connecting lines, altering infusions and checking the urine output, while one of the SHOs, David, wrote up her notes and drug chart on the bedside computer. Linda looked sick. She was sprawled in the bed, with one arm sticking out through the rails and her head thrown to the side. Her eyes were closed and each out-breath was accompanied by a low-pitched groan. There would be no witty asides tonight.

'It's OK, Linda,' Daniel reassured her, 'the consultant is here now.'

Great, no pressure then.

Matt had an echocardiogram (echo, for short) probe on Linda's chest.* Linda's heart was beating fast and hard. One might argue that it should have been beating even harder in the circumstances, but the troponin, a blood marker of heart-muscle damage, had come back as normal. Her heart was not the primary problem.

'Linda,' I called, picking up her hand, 'my name is Jim Down, I'm one of the ICU doctors. We met before, about a year ago. I'm just going to examine you.'

Linda opened her eyes and looked up at me, but she didn't reply. If she did recognize me she was in no mood for small talk. Her skin was clammy to the touch and, despite all the fluid and a hot air blanket, her hands and feet were icy cold. Her chest sounded clear, with just some reduced breath sounds where there was a small amount of fluid around the left lung base, and her oxygen levels were good. She winced when I pressed into her abdomen, but it wasn't rigid as you'd expect if something

---

* The echo is an ultrasound machine that we use to look specifically at heart function. Highly trained technicians can pick up a multitude of subtle pathologies relating to the valves and pressures, but intensivists use it to look at the overall function of the two sides of the heart and for a few other major abnormalities.

catastrophic had happened. I looked all over her body for any infected wounds or ulcers but there was nothing. Her skin was intact and blameless.

'The surgical reg has been and looked at the scan,' Matt told me. 'Nothing to do surgically.'

'Thanks.'

I logged on to the computer and looked through the blood tests. The markers of inflammation/infection were up and the liver and kidneys were struggling, but otherwise there was nothing helpful.

'Anything in the urine?' I asked. As Petros in Chapter 1 had proved, urine infections can make people very sick very quickly.

'Clear.'

I reread the CT scan report and then slumped back into a chair.

'What the hell's going on?' I asked no one in particular.

'Infection from somewhere and then liver decompensation?' Matt suggested. We already knew that Linda's cirrhotic liver coped badly with the added burden of an infection.

'But from where?'

Matt didn't have an answer to that.

'SBP?' I mused.*

'There is some ascites, but not loads.'

'Enough to tap?'

'Sure. I'll do it now.'

---

* Spontaneous bacterial peritonitis: infected fluid within the abdominal cavity. The fluid accumulates because of back pressure from the shrunken cirrhotic liver and can then become infected by bacteria that have leaked through the wall of the bowel. Patients with alcoholic cirrhosis also have reduced immune function so the infection can run wild. It usually happens when there are litres of free fluid in the abdomen, but it is possible with a small volume too.

It was certainly worth sending off a sample. If significantly infected, the fluid would look cloudy or pus-like in the syringe. Mat identified an area of fluid with an ultrasound probe and aspirated 20ml into a syringe. It looked as clear as a freshly poured glass of Chablis, but we sent it to the lab anyway – in hope more than expectation.

Over the next four hours we tried to stabilize Linda. We supported her kidneys and her blood pressure, we sent more samples of sputum, urine and blood to look for infection and we added new antibiotics. Repeat blood tests results were worse, but we were no nearer knowing why. We looked again at the blood flow to the liver with an ultrasound, but it was fine, so eventually I rang my second-on-call consultant colleague for another opinion. He was a bit bleary (by now it was 3.30 a.m.) but also generously uncomplaining as I went through the case and my thoughts. He came up with a couple of things to exclude (dissection of one of the major blood vessels and drug or poison overdose), but otherwise agreed that it was an extremely odd case and that we were doing all the right things.

At 5 a.m. Linda became even more breathless and increasingly drowsy, so we put her to sleep, intubated her and took over her breathing. It was a relief to have ended her immediate suffering and taken control, but the relief was short-lived. Her blood pressure was still low and her lactic-acid level was increasing. We were using a haemofilter, but she was producing the acid faster than the machine could clear it, so I increased the rate of the dialysis and requested a chest X-ray to check the position of the endotracheal tube. The radiographers were busy, so it wasn't until 6.30 a.m. that we got the film and saw that, although the breathing tube was beautifully positioned, there was now a lot of fluid around the left lung. Fluid often accumulates around the lungs of critically ill patients because their blood vessels and tissues become leaky, but it shouldn't have accumulated that quickly. And why was it only on one side?

'Let's drain that,' I said to Matt, a horrible thought crossing my mind for the first time.

'Sure,' he replied. 'Is the clotting OK?'

'No . . . shit! OK, get some FFP into her and Vitamin K and then put a drain in.'

The liver usually synthesizes many of the proteins that make blood clot, but Linda's wasn't producing enough of them, so we needed to top them up with donated plasma (fresh frozen plasma, or FFP) before sticking a big tube into her chest.

It was 8 a.m. before the FFP was defrosted and I had to move my car before it got towed. I phoned Tish on my way across Euston Road, but my daughter Edie answered.

'Where are you?' she asked, getting straight to the point as ever.

'Work, bad night. Are you OK?'

'Tom is really annoying me. He gets, like, *no* homework.'

'Hi, Dad. It's not my fault.'

'Hi, Tom, how are you?'

'Tired.'

'Me too.'

'Fidget brought a dead rat in and then Betty trod on it and smeared blood all over the posh room carpet.'

'God! Is Mum OK?'

'She got quite sweary.'

Fidget (classily named after the spinners) is an exquisite but unbelievably arrogant Maine Coon cat and Betty, a scruffy, gormless Border terrier. They barely acknowledge each other's existence, but between them, run amok.

By the time I got back the chest tube was in and my worst fears had been realized. The fluid coming out this time looked nothing like Chablis. It looked more like gravy. It hadn't accumulated from the lung tissues, it had leaked from the stomach. At some point in the previous three days Linda's vomiting had been so violent that she had ruptured her oesophagus and the contents of her stomach were now leaking into her chest. That was what was making her so ill. The stomach is filled with acid and half-digested food (and alcohol in her case). If that gets into the spaces around the heart and lungs it's not good for you.

'Can you call the upper GI surgeons,' I asked the new day registrar, who was being brought up to speed by Matt. 'Thanks so much, Matt, you should get off home. I'm going to have another look at the CT scan with one of our own radiologists.'

When we reviewed the scan with the new clinical information, it was obvious that the oesophagus was ruptured. There were small pockets of air in the surrounding tissues where there shouldn't have been and we could even make out the hole in the oesophageal wall. It had been missed by the first radiologist and it would be easy for me to blame them, but it was not what we'd asked them to look for. Ruptured oesophagus from vomiting (Boerhaave syndrome) is not uncommon in alcoholics, but the story is usually of sudden, severe chest pain after days of copious violent vomiting, and that wasn't how Linda had presented. She'd had abdominal pain and she hadn't emphasized the vomiting, so I'd assumed that something was going on in her abdomen. She'd also had no problem with her breathing, and her lactic acid level was very high for a Boerhaave. I hadn't thought of it and we hadn't mentioned it on the CT scan request form. I felt awful. I *should* have thought of it.

The treatment of Boerhaave syndrome is to decompress both sides of the leak (with drains in the stomach and chest), to stabilize the patient as we were trying to do, give antibiotics and then if possible either to repair the hole with sutures or to cover it with a stent. By the time the surgeons arrived at 9 a.m. Linda was not fit for an operation. Her liver had taken a big hit and it was all we could do to keep her blood pressure up and clear her lactic acid. The surgeons said they'd put more drains in to control the source of sepsis and then we'd have to watch and wait to see if she improved enough to have definitive surgery. None of us was optimistic.

I updated her family, handed over to my colleague who'd generously offered to cover for a few hours and then slunk off home to get some sleep. But I didn't sleep well.

Linda clung on for the next forty-eight hours. The drains and antibiotics seemed to make some impact and we managed to reduce the support for her blood pressure. Two or three more days of improvement and we might be able to think again about taking her back to the operating theatre, but Linda's liver function was not getting better. Despite support, her blood clotting was still abnormal, her lactic-acid level stubbornly high, and she'd now become jaundiced.

Three nights after her admission I was on call again. Linda was stable when we saw her on the afternoon ward round, but at 10 p.m. Matt called. He was on the last of his four night shifts and Linda was now bleeding, heavily. Fresh blood was coming up out of her mouth and into chest drains and her blood pressure had dropped. I went straight back to the hospital and called in the gastroenterologists, surgeons and radiologists to see what we could do to stop the bleeding. I also called in Linda's family. While we gave blood, fluid and clotting products, the gastroenterologists looked into her stomach with an endoscope and stopped what bleeding they could but there was blood coming from everywhere. The blood vessels were dilated and tortuous due to back pressure from the liver and a couple had ruptured. The gastroenterologists clipped them, but the whole lining of the stomach was also raw and ulcerated. They'd only been able to deal with half of the problem. She wouldn't survive an operation and there was no specific source blood vessel that the radiologists could block. The only thing left to do was give blood and clotting factors and hope that it would stop, but it didn't. Her blood was once again profoundly acidic and she was cold. In these conditions the blood struggles to form clots whatever we give, but we carried on trying. Then, at 4 a.m., her heart flicked into a horrible looking rhythm. It had all been too much and it was time to face the inevitable truth. She was dying. Fifteen minutes later, with her brother and son by the bed, she passed away peacefully in her sleep.

When I'd expressed my condolences to Linda's family I found myself loitering, looking for something more that I could do for them. Anything to make it better, to make amends for what I'd failed to do three nights previously.

'Thank you for trying,' they said.

I went and reviewed a couple of other patients who might need to come to the ICU and then at 5 a.m. I went home. But I was not all right. I felt guilty, anxious and stupid. I was convinced that I was responsible for Linda's death. I had the strong impression that one of the senior nurses thought I could have done better on the first night and, although I tried to persuade myself that it wouldn't have changed the outcome, a part of me agreed with her.

Had I lost my clinical acumen?

I'd certainly lost my confidence.

Over the next few weeks the events of that first night went round and round in my head. I tried to blame the Australian radiologists, but I had asked them to look for the wrong things. Over and over again I kept asking myself why I didn't think of Boerhaave. I pictured Linda with her sly smile, making pithy remarks the year before, and as I did so, the guilt and self-loathing welled up in me. I could think about nothing else. I couldn't sleep, I didn't know what to say to my children and I couldn't see the point of anything. I couldn't remember how to enjoy things. I didn't think I deserved happiness. I kept imagining what her brother and son were doing now. How were they feeling? Were they coping? When I went for a walk and saw people laughing and messing about, I felt angry. Why were they happy? Did they not know that she was dead?

My anxiety level rose and fell and rose again. For a while it would feel manageable, but then something would remind me of what had happened and it would start to build, a knot ratcheting tighter and tighter in my stomach. I felt sick as intrusive negative thoughts bombarded my consciousness. I could explain to Tish what was happening quite rationally, but I couldn't stop it. The terrible thoughts just kept coming and, with them, panic.

You are not good enough. You should have done better. You've been getting away with it for years. You need to work harder, or give up. It's time to face it, you're just not up to the job.

I picked the case apart with several colleagues. They all concluded (or at least said they concluded) that I had done a decent job. Linda had been incredibly sick and, once her liver started to fail, she'd collapsed like a house of cards. It was an unusual presentation and the scan had been reported as normal. Even if I'd thought of Boerhaave, it wouldn't have made any difference. The die was cast. While they were saying it I believed them and felt better, but soon the doubts crept back in.

Tish was endlessly supportive. She was patient and understanding and tried to persuade me that I was being far too hard on myself.

'You went straight in and you spent the whole night at the bedside, doing everything you could to make her better. You talked it through with your colleague, the surgeons reviewed, the scan was reported as normal – what else could you have done? Listen to your colleagues!'

My dad said the same.

Even the children tried to make me feel better by temporarily refraining from walloping each other around the head at every opportunity and going to brush their teeth when I asked.

No one else was worried about how I'd managed the patient, but people were starting to worry about me. As one of the registrars pointed out at the time, I had done my best, but it had not been enough, and in my mind that was almost worse. Would Linda have survived if someone *better* had been on call? I spoke to more colleagues, who reassured me that they'd have done nothing differently. Generously, they talked about patients who haunted their thoughts, but still I felt awful.

I knew that my reaction was extreme and that I was not really to blame, but I couldn't change the way I felt. People suggested that the way I was feeling was the result of a culmination of stressors that weren't related to Linda and I could see that that made sense. I had always been vulnerable to anxiety and I had just been through a year of working in a Covid ICU. During that time I'd also hardly seen my mother, whose dementia was progressing rapidly. It had been heartbreaking to watch from afar her personality fade and to hear stories of the daily struggles of my father, culminating eventually in her admission to a nursing home.

I agreed that Linda was probably just the straw that broke the camel's back, but it didn't feel like that. It felt all consuming, overwhelming and catastrophic. The one thing I did know was that I wanted to recover. I never felt suicidal and I always wanted to feel normal again, so I threw everything I could at the problem.

The ICU clinical director was very sympathetic and suggested that I contact the staff psychological service. I'd never even considered doing that in the past. I knew that it existed, but I couldn't imagine a scenario in which I'd call them. What would I tell them? Who would they tell? Would they really understand and what could they actually do? The risks had always seemed far greater than the small chance of benefit, but now I felt I had nothing to lose. I set up a video meeting with a staff psychologist and then followed it up with face-to-face appointments. She was practical and reassuring. She taught me breathing and tapping techniques* for when things were particularly bad and then we did sessions of EMDR (eye movement desensitizing and reprocessing). It's a technique used in the treatment of post-traumatic stress disorder (PTSD) in which the stressful event is recalled while performing particular eye movements to reprocess it in the brain (or something like that). I didn't really understand it, but it seemed to help. In her room I felt safe, and I remember thinking, *I'm fine, I'm wasting your time*, but as soon as I left, I felt anxious again and returned to hours of ruminating on the what ifs, despite my best intentions. I kept picturing Linda in Bed 16 that first night, groaning, exhausted and helpless.

Eventually, I spoke to a close friend from medical school who had become a psychiatrist. It was impressive to hear the way he moved subtly from a chat between mates to professional assessment. Within ten minutes he'd concluded that I was probably depressed, so I called my GP. I've never met my GP, but she was brilliant on the telephone consultation and agreed with my

---

* The tapping technique involved crossing my hands across my chest with thumbs interlinked in a 'butterfly formation' and rhythmically tapping my collar bones when the anxiety became overwhelming. Much like box breathing (breathing in for four seconds, holding for four seconds, out for four seconds and holding for four seconds) it reduced the acute anxiety and temporarily broke the cycle of negative thoughts.

friend. She suggested that I combine the talking therapy with antidepressants.

'You might feel more anxious to begin with, but try to keep going with them,' she said. 'If you can. It will pass.'

Never was a truer word spoken. For the first ten days on antidepressants I was hit by waves of anxiety. It was a new and unfamiliar sensation, because it wasn't focused on anything. Instead I was enveloped by a free-floating, but nevertheless overpowering sensation of angst that made me want to curl up into a ball and groan.

My colleagues covered or backed up my on-calls and both the anaesthetic and intensive care departments were fantastically supportive. They allowed me all the time off I needed to recover, but I couldn't decide whether to stay at home ruminating and potentially upsetting the children or brave work, where I felt anxious and paranoid. The ICU had become a monster. It felt as if danger lurked in every corner, as if every patient would catch me out. Just swiping in through the front doors, where I'd been completely at home for fifteen years, I felt fearful and stressed. I thought everyone was looking at me and judging or pitying me. I assumed that the trainee doctors and the nurses had lost confidence in my judgement and would quietly double-check my decisions in the future. Perhaps I wouldn't be able to make decisions. Perhaps the patients and relatives would pick up on my anxiety. I made a mental list of alternative careers. Could I do something useful on my father-in-law's farm? No, I quickly concluded.

An actor friend, who has suffered from anxiety and depression that manifest as stage fright and insomnia, suggested cold-water swimming. He swims in our local lido throughout the year and raves about its benefits, so Tish and I joined him. It was early May, and the water temperature was 13°C: manageable, but much colder than we were used to. I had always scoffed at the cold-water swimming brigade (probably because I am a terrible swimmer even in warm water), but I was prepared to try anything. After one session, Tish thought better of it, but I was addicted. I wore a wetsuit top to begin with, but halfway through I took it off and relished the tingle of the water against my skin. For the first time since that night in the hospital three weeks previously, my mind cleared. I was fully focused on keeping my head above the freezing water and it was thrilling. I stayed in for forty minutes and then spent an hour and a half shivering next to a radiator. Warming up was as good as getting cold.

For six weeks I ducked out of all social events. I was terrified by the prospect of having to make conversation and convinced that I had nothing to say. I found it difficult enough to concentrate on what my family were saying over the dinner table. My social calendar was not exactly overflowing with commitments, but I missed two very close friends' birthdays and the delayed celebration lunch for the publication of my first book. I had been looking forward to all three gatherings, but now I couldn't face seeing anyone.

In mid-June, Tish and I were invited for supper at my actor friend and his wife's house. We'd arranged it in April and they were one of the few couples that I felt relaxed talking to, albeit mainly at the swimming pool. Intermittently I was beginning to feel slightly better so, at their behest, I agreed to go. A famous actor, one of my son's heroes, had also been invited, so if we'd pulled out I'd never live it down. When the night arrived, I felt relatively stable, so I girded my loins, gripped Tish's arm and we went. I had stopped drinking alcohol, so I drove, and as we rang the doorbell I thought I might well be back in the car and on the way home within an hour. I felt nervous at first and then probably overcompensated by talking too much and too loudly, but soon I relaxed and two hours later I realized that I was OK. I was laughing and joking and I hadn't thought about the case for over an hour. I was enjoying myself. I can still remember the exact moment of thinking that.

People say that the pills give you space. They allow you to regain some perspective and to exert a degree of control over your thoughts and emotions. That was how it felt to me. For the next week or two I felt optimistic. I was sleeping better, eating better and functioning better at work. The children had given up tiptoeing around me and the noise level at home had definitely returned to normal. But sometimes the anxiety crept back in. Someone asked if we could discuss Linda's case at one of our mortality and morbidity meetings and I felt the panic rise up. I had gone over and over it already, far more than was healthy, and there was nothing else I could learn, but I knew it had to be done. I just couldn't face talking about it in public. It was then that I realized how fragile my mental health was. A few days later, though, I rallied again and I have cautiously been moving forward ever since. I am under the care of a wonderful psychiatrist; I took a short course of cognitive behavioural therapy and I am still taking antidepressants. I am lucky. I feel well again, but I am aware that it could all go wrong at any time, and if it does I want to be in the best possible state to deal with it.

I still go to the lido every morning. After the first three weeks I bit the bullet and bought a year's pass. When the temperature hit 10°C I purchased gloves, boots and a hat, but I'm still not wearing a wetsuit. It's January as I write (4°C today), and every morning I join the same ten or fifteen people waiting in the dark for the pool to open at 7 a.m. They are a friendly, funny bunch who take the piss constantly, but they also have each other's backs. When I finally caught Covid and missed ten days, I received an email from a fellow swimmer. It was just one line, sent at 6.55 a.m.: *All OK? Not seen you at the lido for ages.*

Most of them have been coming for years, decades even, but there's no machismo or one-upmanship. Sometimes I wonder what made each of them start. I am still not a strong swimmer (breast stroke all the way), and I regularly take lungfuls of water, but like the rest of them, I'm addicted.

Conclusion

My relationship with the job has changed over the years. My view of what ICU is and what it should be has definitely evolved, but ICU has also changed me.

When I started out, I assumed that I would become wiser and more confident as my career progressed. I looked forward to being the doctor who was never ruffled, who'd seen it all before and whom younger colleagues would phone when they didn't know what to do. I have become wiser, I think, certainly more thoughtful, but not necessarily more confident. For a few years after becoming a consultant, my self-belief grew. I established myself, settled into the role and played to my strengths, but in the last few years the job has gradually worn away at my defences and exposed underlying frailties. For a while there was still enough armour in place for me to carry on and pretend to both the world and myself that I was fine, but deep down I knew that my vulnerabilities were moving ever closer to the surface. I was becoming more anxious, more risk averse and more difficult to live with. Covid accelerated the process and in 2021 it all came to a head. My defences were finally, undeniably breached and I had to stop, reset and start again. After twenty-five years the pressures of ICU and anaesthesia had become too much. It was frightening to acknowledge, but compared to many I was lucky.

Doctors may have a better life expectancy than the general population (even than other people from social class 1), but their risk of suicide is higher. Bullying, complaints, investigations of practice, high physical and mental demand, uncontrollable long hours, shift patterns, working at night, isolation and rigorous postgraduate exams are all risk factors and, unsurprisingly, some specialities are more risky than others. Anaesthesia and intensive care are well known to be high-risk specialities; the question is why? Why do we have such high rates of death from liver cirrhosis and both accidental and deliberate drug overdose? Why are our rates of substance abuse higher than those of most doctors?

Anaesthesia in particular is a peculiar area of medicine. Anaesthetists do not make people better; but with every anaesthetic we can make them a lot worse. Approximately half of the population believe we are not medically qualified and the better we are at the job, the more our skill is overlooked and the more invisible we become. In both anaesthesia and ICU we do not have control over (or sometimes even prior information about) which patients we will be looking after and often our only power is to decide that the risks of proceeding outweigh the benefits and say no, which can be very unpopular with both patients and colleagues. But when we say yes it is our responsibility to keep the patients safe.

This 'authority to responsibility gap' is often quoted when describing the relative stress of different jobs. Having the authority and control to match your level of responsibility is important. If a bus driver is told that she must drive her bus full of children up an icy mountain road or lose her job, she is likely to feel extremely stressed. Her options are to refuse and be sacked or take the risk, drive really carefully and hope for the best. Her responsibility couldn't be higher but her authority does not match it. If she planned the bus trips and decided when and whether she set off up the mountain her responsibility would still be as high, arguably higher, but it would be matched by authority and her stress levels would be lower. She would have genuine control over the decision.

We are not sacked for cancelling cases or refusing ICU admissions, but we are acutely aware that, every day, we take on the responsibility for our patients' lives. There is often little warning or discussion of the risk profile and sometimes the relevant information is incomplete. Most anaesthetists do not meet their patients until the morning of surgery and intensivists often only find out about patients who are deteriorating on the wards in the middle of the night, when the patient is *in extremis* and there is no time for a rational discussion about the appropriateness of ICU admission.

The vast majority of cases are manageable, but routinely we give drugs that both stop people breathing and drop their blood pressure. In a few patients, one or other of those is life threatening, and the constant low-level niggle that one of those patients might turn up on your list or in your ICU the next day can progress into an unhealthy state of mind.

Doctors describe the sensation when it goes wrong as a gut punch. I am not claiming that this is unique to anaesthesia and intensive care, or even to medicine, but there *is* something unique about taking a person who is sitting talking to you and, in a matter of minutes, rendering them helpless, unconscious and paralysed.

When I had been doing the job for six months one of my bosses, the senior consultant in the department and a nationally revered figure, asked me how it was going.

'Well,' I replied, eager to please, 'I think I've got the hang of it.'

'That's just when it will slap you in the face,' he replied.

By 2021 I had become fixated on what could go wrong. I was sure that a gut punch was coming and I think that, subconsciously, I was willing it on, to get it over and done with. On some level I felt that I deserved it. My reaction to Linda's death was disproportionate and irrational. It was a tragic case, but I had done my best and I think that I reacted as I did because I was waiting for it. Above the surface I was trying to ward it off, taking extra precautions, checking and double-checking and getting lots of second opinions from colleagues, but all the time beneath the waves I was just waiting. Somewhere deep inside me was the notion that I couldn't avoid it. It was my turn and it was coming. I didn't realize this at the time, and it was only when I had to examine my fears and anxieties later, in therapy, that I understood what had been going on. As I ran through the case for the umpteenth time with a couple of very patient colleagues, one of them put their finger on it.

'How do you deal with uncertainty?' he asked simply.

That was my problem. My obsession with disaster grew out of my inability to accept uncertainty. I wanted to eliminate risk and make myself bulletproof because people's lives were at stake, but I couldn't. Having this one case go badly wasn't going to make the future safer any more than Baldrick writing his name on a bullet was going to stop him being shot. I needed to learn to live with the uncertainty. I wasn't going to become cavalier, but I had to strike a balance. One in five patients who come to the ICU die. It's a high-risk environment. Most of the deaths are unavoidable, but not all. The clinical decisions we make often have no right answers, but they still have profound implications. Inevitably, that leaves us with a lot of what ifs, and that was something I had to come to terms with.

For now, at least, I have.

But how has my view of ICU changed over the years?

I think ICU is a confusing place. At first glance, it's all highly technical: big, bright, beeping machines. The atmosphere is clean and clinical, the equipment shiny and intimidating and the staff highly skilled and professional. The stereotypical ICU patient was fit and well two weeks ago, but has now been hit by catastrophe. The young man who crashed his motorbike at eighty miles an hour, the teenager with the florid rash and black fingers and toes of meningococcal septicaemia, the forty-year-old mother of two who collapsed when a weak blood vessel in her brain popped without warning, or the naive festival-goer who reacted badly to a cocktail of party drugs. Each of these patients has been pushed to beyond what their bodies can deal with. Their physiology can no longer support itself and the role of ICU is obvious; it must step in, take over the functions of their vital organs and keep them alive.

These cases are the stuff of TV dramas – the flawed but good-hearted protagonist with so much potential, whose life is in the balance. The only question on anyone's lips is, 'Will they make it?' While there is a chance, the medics will do everything. (Of course they will, goddammit!)

But in reality ICU is about much more than this. Every case is nuanced, and few of the issues are black and white. Most of the people who come our way are no longer spring chickens and many are already living with chronic health problems and limited physiological reserve. Even if they did start out fit, their potential to return to that state is often limited by whatever has happened to them. We might be able to keep them alive, but at what cost? How much brain function will the mother with the popped blood vessel get back? Will the man who crashed his motorbike ever be able to care for himself again? Will the child with meningococcal sepsis be left without hands and feet? On TV it's all about whether our hero will 'make it', but in real life that's only one of several questions.

So, our ability to keep people alive artificially in this high-tech twilight zone makes us re-examine some fundamental questions. What gives life meaning? What makes it worth living? How much suffering is too much and how much function is enough? Is it binary or is there a continuous scale? Should one quality of life be judged as more valuable than another? All these questions inevitably lead on to another – who should decide?

My answer used to be that ICU was only for people who had a decent chance of returning to a good quality of life – not quite the heroes from TV, but not a million miles away. I made well-intentioned but imperfect judgements about that potential every day, and I felt that it was my duty to put up barriers against dubious admissions. There was an unspoken code: the ologists made the case for bringing their patients to ICU and I evaluated it. It was their unofficial job to persuade me. Sometimes they did, sometimes I changed their minds, but occasionally we arrived at an impasse. The oncologist might firmly believe that two or three days on the ventilator would turn their cancer patient round and give them several good months, while I was convinced that once ventilated they'd inevitably die miserably in ICU.

In those circumstances I explained to the patient and/or relatives that ICU was a tough, painful, unpleasant, noisy and frightening place. Were they sure it was what they or their loved one would want? That sounds brutal, but I wasn't unkind. I was desperately worried about filling my beds with hopeless cases that would lie there gloomily for weeks and then succumb. In many ways, I argued, the easy option was to take everyone, but the ICU wasn't a destination, it was only a stepping stone back to health. If you wouldn't be able to step off that stone, then you shouldn't step onto it. By the same logic, when a case already on the unit became hopeless, I saw it as my duty to apprise the relatives and the home team of the situation and palliate that patient as soon as was compassionately possible. My responsibility was to marshal the use of our very expensive stepping stone, however harsh that sometimes seemed.

But then, gradually, something in me shifted. I'd never found these decisions easy because it was often impossible to judge which patients were inappropriate. But I'd always accepted that decisions had to be made, and that I was doing my best in an imperfect world, until I started to notice things that made me wonder whether that was entirely true. I realized that when someone I knew personally or particularly admired came through ICU, it affected my decision making. I was just that little bit more aware of what their loss would mean, so I was fractionally more likely to give them the benefit of the doubt and treat them for longer. It didn't mean that I was necessarily giving them superior treatment – I might just be prolonging their suffering – but it did mean that I was appraising more than just the physiology. The perceived value of the patient's life, not just its quality, was influencing my decisions. I worked hard to remain impartial and to resist these impulses, but they were still there.

I also noticed that I was affected by the attitude of relatives. If a family were particularly aggressive or litigious, I was more likely to acquiesce to their demands than if they were accommodating and polite. That's not an easy thing to admit, and again I fought against it, but still, on occasion, it happened.

And at around the same time it dawned on me that, despite my best efforts, I wasn't necessarily always getting to the heart of what the patients really thought or wanted. When I explained the grisly details of ICU they often agreed that it was not for them, only to reverse their decision having talked to their distraught children or optimistic oncologist. For years I viewed the conclusions of those subsequent conversations as either coerced or unrealistic, but now I wasn't sure.

And I began to imagine a member of my own family in the patients' position. Was I really sure that I'd always accept my own advice if it was my dad in the bed? What about if *I* was in the bed?

I thought that, 95 per cent of the time, I would, because I was an experienced ICU doctor and I was making careful, considered decisions, but still, perhaps I was being a bit too rigid in my view of what ICU could and should do. Perhaps it wasn't just for people with the potential, desire and drive to get back to a full and active life. Of course, we all needed to remain realistic, but that didn't mean we couldn't use the beds more creatively. If we had the space, we could admit borderline cases for a 'trial' of ICU support on the understanding that if they didn't respond we'd move to palliation. We could take patients explicitly for lower-level support such as CPAP while they considered their future wishes, said goodbye to loved ones or put their affairs in order and, in certain circumstances, it could even be a place to come to die.

These days I take a lot of people I am not sure about. The likelihood might be that they'll not do well, but if they have a chance and they're keen, then I embrace my doubt and bring them in. The downside, of course, is that more people suffer unpleasant ICU intervention only to succumb anyway, but that's a price that I am (judiciously) prepared to pay, because it is often impossible to know categorically in advance whether a specific patient will benefit from ICU. In the end it is a judgement, so, when we have enough beds, I use ICU for anyone I think might benefit, whatever form that benefit takes.

But should I be given this freedom?

ICU is expensive. Every occupied bed costs the taxpayer £1,500 to £2,000 per day. If a new drug came along that cost as much it would be evaluated by the National Institute for Health and Care Excellence before being approved for use within the NHS. The manufacturer would have to prove that it delivered value for money in terms of added quality-adjusted life years or similar and the patient eligibility criteria would be strict. ICU has never undergone that level of scrutiny. I can use my beds for whomever I want, but a public health-care system should have equity and value for money at its core and many would argue that some of the people I admit are not good use of taxpayer's money. Another intensivist on another day might choose not to take them, so the care isn't necessarily equitable either.

So what should the future of ICU look like? We could throw endless money at the problem and give patients and their relatives autonomy to demand whatever they want. I am told that there are private hospitals in other countries with rows of patients in persistent vegetative state who have been ventilated for decades. At the other extreme the government could dictate that ICU beds be allocated only to patients with certain conditions, physiological reserve and quality of life. Or we could continue to muddle through as we do now and allow experienced doctors to make what they think is the best decision in collaboration with the patients and families.

A final option would be to combine all three. The government could draw up guidelines with scope for clinician interpretation and a process by which relatives can appeal. That would require us to acknowledge that there is rationing and that we actually follow a benefit-based rather than fairness-based ethical framework.*

I love having the autonomy to use ICU beds in the way I see fit, but I can see that the money might be better spent on a new drug, preventive medicine or improved mental health services. ICU is only a small cog in the NHS machine and we are duty bound to examine what we achieve. The distribution of ICU beds is currently undertaken on an ad hoc, day-to-day

* A fairness-based ethical framework suggests that anyone who has a reasonable chance of benefit from an intervention should be offered it, whereas a benefit-based framework determines those who will benefit most and prioritizes them.

basis – we've got this many beds today and this many staff, so we'll give them to these patients. Perhaps if there were guidelines, we might focus this expensive resource on those most likely to benefit.

But then there are people like John, Jonathan and Susannah.

John was a ninety-four-year-old retired judge with Covid pneumonia whom we admitted for high-flow oxygen and some blood-pressure support. I had to seek his consent to drain some fluid from around his lungs to help his breathing, so I scribbled down his details and the procedure on a consent form and thrust it into his hands. We had discussed the risks and I expected him to sign without a second glance (most people do, even before major surgery), but not a bit of it. He took the form and began to study it. Assuming he was looking for the place to sign, I pointed out the dotted line, but he waved me away with a, 'Yes, yes, I know,' so I stood back and waited patiently. A couple of minutes later he beckoned me over.

'You've not ticked this box. Is there a reason for that?' I followed his finger to an obscure box on the form that I'd never even noticed before.

'Sorry about that, er . . . sure, let me have a look.'

Fifteen minutes later I had a much more detailed understanding of our consent forms and one carefully signed by him. He smiled up at me and said, 'Right, let's get on with it,' and we did.

With the drain in, there was a small chance he'd improve enough to get home, but we also decided to treat him on the ICU because he desperately wanted to write a particular academic paper before he died (UCH is a teaching hospital, we love research). I suggested that he could write it on a laptop while on the unit and he leapt at the idea. All the information was in his head and he was bursting to write it down. He, his eighty-seven-year-old wife and I agreed that intubation and ventilation would be a step too far, but while he could still breathe for himself he was keen to keep fighting. Covid visiting restrictions were still in place, but we were relatively quiet so I offered his wife an extra visit the next day.

'Well, I don't think he'll . . .' She hesitated and turned to her husband. 'Would you like me to visit tomorrow, dear?'

'What? Oh, no no no,' he replied. 'I'll be working tomorrow, stick to Sunday.'

She turned back to me and smiled. He began work on his paper and then a few days later he died peacefully in his sleep.

Jonathan was twenty-four years old and suffered from Duchenne muscular dystrophy, an incurable disease in which the muscles become progressively weaker through childhood. Most Duchenne's patients are in a wheelchair by the age of twelve and die in their later teens of respiratory muscle failure. Jonathan was wheelchair-bound and required ventilatory support overnight via a tight-fitting mask, and the support of carers several times every day, but he had recently graduated from university, where he'd managed to live in the halls of residence.

In November 2011 Jonathan's stomach twisted, lost its blood supply and necrosed. Jonathan became extremely sick very quickly and went for emergency surgery to have it removed, his gullet tied off and a feeding tube inserted into his small bowel. He came back to ICU looking awful. He was fully ventilated, on a lot of drugs to keep his blood pressure up and immediately needed support for his kidneys. We all thought his outlook was hopeless and prepared his family for the worst but, remarkably, he improved. His blood pressure stabilized and his kidneys kicked back in. The only problem left was his breathing, and after a few weeks it became clear that he was never going to be free of the tracheostomy or ventilator. He was also never going to eat again (he was a foody, usually persuading his carers to cook even when his fellow students were living off takeaways) and he had already exceeded his life expectancy, so it felt uncomfortable to put him through ongoing intensive care to no end. Except that he wanted us to. Even if he could never get out of the unit, he wanted to carry on. He was awake, he was determined, he had capacity and life was worth living. I don't remember him ever complaining about his lot.

It might look awful to an outsider and seem futile in the face of a terminal disease, but it wasn't to Jonathan – so we carried on. When he got an infection we increased his support and gave him antibiotics, and by the summer of 2012 he was well enough to do short trips out of the hospital. A highlight was when our nurse consultant and one of the physiotherapists took him (with his ventilator) for a day trip to watch the Paralympics.

After more than 300 days on the ICU, and against all the odds, Jonathan went home. He took a ventilator with him and required twenty-four-hour care, but he made it back to his parents' house and lived another three years. Life was tougher than before, and frustrating at times, but he continued to enjoy films, music, his PlayStation and Man United.

Susannah was a forty-year-old mother of two with terminal breast cancer who was breathless on the oncology ward with a chest infection. On learning of her prognosis six months earlier, she had quit her high-powered job in the Civil Service and devoted the time she had left to her daughters. She and her husband took them on a road trip through California, camped in the Scottish Highlands and canoed down the Dordogne river. When she became weaker and could no longer go out, she wrote a journal telling them everything she had learnt about life, mainly from all the mistakes she had made.

If she was afraid of death, she didn't let it show, but her one overriding wish was to die at home, with her family and her dogs, so we admitted her. We gave her blood-pressure support and antibiotics, drained fluid from her abdomen and chest and asked our palliative care colleagues to set up a package to get her home. She spent three days with us on ICU so that she could spend one more day in her own home, surrounded by all the people she loved, before she died.

I hate the idea of not being able to offer these patients the support they want. I can also see that perhaps we should be striving to come up with national guidance about how we use ICU. Fortunately, such guidance will be fiendishly difficult, if not impossible to write, and then get agreed, so it is highly unlikely to be produced before I retire. I just hope that it doesn't come out when I'm a frail ninety-four-year-old with a research project to finish, hoping for an ICU bed.

Glossary

ACS   Acute coronary syndrome. Blockage to one of the arteries supplying the heart. Otherwise known as a myocardial infarction or a heart attack.

AF   Atrial Fibrillation. A common heart arrhythmia in which the small chambers of the heart (the atria) do not contract in an organized way, reducing the efficiency and stability of the heartbeat.

Anaphylaxis   A potentially life-threatening form of allergic reaction characterized by rash, wheezing and a fall in blood pressure.

Antibodies   Proteins produced by the immune system that recognize and bind to unwanted substances in the body to help eliminate them.

Apnoea   Absence of breathing.

Arterial line   A cannula that sits in the artery of a patient and is used for continuous blood pressure monitoring and blood sampling.

Blood cultures   A test to look for bacteria or other infections within the bloodstream.

Blood gas   A bedside blood test that measures the levels of oxygen, carbon dioxide, acid, haemoglobin, lactate, sodium and potassium in the blood.

'Bloods'   Colloquial term for blood tests used to measure blood cell counts, electrolytes and other molecules in the blood.

Clerking	The initial medical assessment of a patient, comprising history, examination, investigations and differential diagnosis.
CPAP	Continuous positive airway pressure. Constant positive pressure applied to the mouth and nose via a mask or hood (like sticking your head out of the car window on the motorway). CPAP is used to open the airways, open the lungs or to reduce the strain on the heart.
CPR	Cardiopulmonary resuscitation. The use of chest compressions and artificial breaths to maintain a flow of oxygen to the brain when the heart has stopped, while efforts are made to restart it.
Creatinine	A product of muscle metabolism that is cleared from the blood by the kidneys and so acts as a marker of kidney function.
Crepitations	Often shortened to creps or crackles. A sound (like a crisp packet being scrunched) heard in the chest when the air spaces contain fluid and open and close through the breath cycle.
Cricoid	A ring of cartilage around the trachea, situated just below the Adam's apple.
CRP	C reactive protein. A non-specific blood marker of inflammation.
Diastolic blood pressure	*See* Systolic blood pressure.
Diuretics	Drugs that increase urine output, often used for fluid retention, heart failure or high blood pressure.
DNR	Do not resuscitate (also referred to as DNACPR – do not attempt cardio-pulmonary resuscitation).
ECG	Electrocardiogram. A recording of the electrical activity in the heart via sensors on the skin.

	ECGs detect the rhythm and rate of the heart and identify abnormalities such as heart attacks.
ED	Emergency Department (used to be called Accident and Emergency and before that Casualty).
Fasciotomies	Surgical incisions made to reduce the pressure in a compartment of the body (usually in the limbs).
FY1, FY2	See SHO.
GCS	Glasgow Coma Scale. An objective grading of conscious level. The lowest score is 3/15 when the patient does not respond at all to a painful stimulus, up to 15/15 when the patient is awake and orientated.
Gentamicin (gent)	A powerful antibiotic that is often added to an IV drip when patients are very unwell.
GMC	General Medical Council. A body that maintains the official register of medical practitioners. Its primary function is to protect the safety of the public by controlling entry to the register and suspending or removing practitioners when necessary.
Gram neg bacteria	A type of bacteria that stain in a particular way under a microscope.
Haematologists	Doctors specializing in disorders of the blood.
Haemofilter	ICU dialysis-type machine that stands five feet tall and takes over from the kidneys when they stop functioning adequately. Also referred to as the 'filter'.
Hypotension	Lower than normal blood pressure.
ICU	Intensive Care Unit, sometimes referred to as Intensive Therapy Unit or Critical Care Unit. Also referred to here as 'the unit'.
IM	Intra-muscular. Injection of medication directly into a muscle, which is particularly useful in an emergency when there is no intravenous access.

Immunosuppression	Reduced function of the immune system, caused either by disease or by drugs, which reduces the body's ability to fight infection.
Inflammation	The response of the body to injury or infection, manifest as warmth, redness, swelling and tenderness. It is part of the healing process but, when dysregulated can become chronic and harmful.
Intubation	The process of inserting an endotracheal tube. Referred to colloquially as 'tubing'.
Jaundice	Yellow discoloration of the skin and eyes as a result of high bilirubin levels in the blood. Bilirubin is a product of red blood cell breakdown which is altered in the liver and then excreted in the bile. Jaundice occurs when there is liver disease, blockage of bile drainage or excessive red blood cell breakdown.
Lactate	The ionized form of lactic acid. It is usually present at a low level in the blood but builds up in the presence of anaerobic metabolism (when inadequate oxygen is reaching the tissues) or when the liver fails.
Laryngoscope	An instrument with a curved blade that is placed over the tongue to give a view of the larynx and allow intubation.
Leukaemia	Cancer that starts in blood-forming tissue, such as the bone marrow, and then releases abnormal malignant blood cells into the circulation.
Lymphoma	Cancer of the lymphatic system, which includes lymph glands, the spleen, the thymus gland and bone marrow.
MCS	Minimally conscious state. A state of minimal or inconsistent awareness. The patient may have

periods when they can communicate or obey commands.

MRI — Magnetic Resonance Imaging. A type of scan that uses a strong magnetic field and radio waves (but no radiations) to produce detailed cross-sectional images of the body.

Palliation — Treatments to relieve the symptoms of life-threatening diseases but not to cure them.

PCR — Polymerase chain reaction. A technique that amplifies a section of DNA. It is used, among other things, to identify the presence of pathogens in different fluid samples.

PEP — Post-exposure prophylaxis. Medication given after potential exposure to a pathogen (particularly HIV) to prevent development of the disease.

Platelets — Blood cells involved in the formation of blood clots.

PVS — Persistent vegetative state. A post-coma state of wakefulness but without awareness or cognition.

Registrar — Senior trainee doctor (between SHO and consultant). Officially now referred to as a Speciality Trainee (ST) 3–8. (The nomenclature changes regularly.)

Resus — Resuscitation room in the Emergency Department.

Rigor — Shivering (often severe) associated with a fever.

SBP — Spontaneous bacterial peritonitis. Infected fluid within the abdominal cavity, common in patients with cirrhosis of the liver.

Sepsis — Infection in the bloodstream that leads to tissue damage and organ failure.

SHO — Senior house officer. Junior-level trainee doctor now officially referred to as FY (Foundation

Year) 2 and Speciality Trainees (ST) 1–2 (although slightly different in different specialities and changing all the time). FY1s used to be known as junior house officers.

Shock   Low blood pressure leading to inadequate blood and oxygen supply to vital organs. Caused usually by heart dysfunction, overwhelming infection/inflammation, bleeding, anaphylaxis or spinal cord injury.

SpO$_2$/oxygen sats   The percentage of haemoglobin (the molecule that carries oxygen in the blood) that is saturated with oxygen. Arterial blood is usually > 96% saturated and venous blood 75%; 25% of the oxygen is extracted by the tissues.

Systolic blood pressure   The peak figure of blood pressure during a heartbeat (the lower figure being diastolic blood pressure, between beats – when the heart is relaxed while refilling).

Tachycardia   A heart rate of greater than a hundred beats per minute.

Tachypnoea   Rapid breathing at greater than twenty breaths per minute.

UCH   University College Hospital. Part of University College London Hospitals (UCLH) NHS Trust.

Ultrasound   A non-invasive machine for looking at tissues and organs within the body using high-energy sound waves. Examples include prenatal foetal scans and echocardiograms that look at the foetus and the structure and function of the heart, respectively.

VHF   Viral haemorrhagic fever. A group of severe viral

infections (including Ebola) that can affect multiple organs in the body and lead to bleeding and sometimes death.

White blood cells   Blood cells involved in inflammation and fighting infection.

Acknowledgements

Thank you first to all the patients and relatives of patients who allowed me to include them in this book – you all taught me so much. Thanks also to my fantastic colleagues at UCH, particularly in ICU, anaesthetics and theatres. You've also taught me quite a lot and I wouldn't want to work anywhere else.

Thank you to Rik Thomas, David Brealey, Monty Mythen, Kate Mythen, Viki Mitchell, Mo Thavasothy, Marie Healy, Sam Clarke, Marina Litvinenko, David Howell, Merlin Hyman, Katy Hyman, Baroness Julia Neuberger, Andrew Mcleod, Sahiba Sethi, Sean Housley, Marina Houseley, Laura Price and John Dick for reading and editing early drafts and for all your generosity and encouragement.

I am indebted to the wonderful, wise and endlessly generous Georgia Garrett for her guidance, patience and humour. A huge thank you to my brilliant editors, Jamie Birkett, Tom Killingbeck, Celia Buzuk and Emma Brown at Viking for carefully bashing this book into shape and to copy editor Trevor Horwood for your extraordinary knowledge and attention to detail. Many thanks also to Jane Gentle and Rosie Safaty at Viking and to Julia Connolly for the brilliant cover design.

Thank you to the 7 a.m. mob at the Lido for keeping me sane and smiling and to Giles Constable, Tom Estcourt, Lisa Monaghan, Tim Bonnici, John Goldstone, Elliot Levey, Emma Loach, Geoff Bellingan, Irene Bouras, Kirstie Macpherson, Jamie Smart, James Holding and Jane Marshall for seeing me through a difficult time.

Thank you to my wonderful family, Peter Down, Mark Down and Caroline Filippin (and Fi and Cristian) and to Mum – I miss you every day. Finally, eternal thanks to Edie, Tom and my wife Tish. This book is for you.